四川大学华西医院

实用新冠肺炎

汉英词汇速查手册

SCU West China Hospital
Chinese-English Notebook
for COVID-19

主编/谢　红　廖明恒　卿　平
主审/程南生　曾　勇

四川大学出版社

项目策划：张　晶　刘　畅　周　艳
责任编辑：刘　畅　周　艳
责任校对：余　芳
封面设计：墨创文化
责任印制：王　炜

图书在版编目（CIP）数据

四川大学华西医院实用新冠肺炎汉英词汇速查手册 / 谢红，廖明恒，卿平主编．— 成都：四川大学出版社，2020.5

ISBN 978-7-5614-7849-3

Ⅰ．①四…　Ⅱ．①谢…　②廖…　③卿…　Ⅲ．①日冕形病毒－病毒病－肺炎－词汇－手册－汉、英　Ⅳ．①R563.1-62

中国版本图书馆 CIP 数据核字（2020）第 069371 号

书名　四川大学华西医院实用新冠肺炎汉英词汇速查手册

Sichuan Daxue Huaxi Yiyuan Shiyong Xinguan Feiyan Han-Ying Cihui Sucha Shouce

主　　编	谢　红　廖明恒　卿　平
出　　版	四川大学出版社
地　　址	成都市一环路南一段 24 号（610065）
发　　行	四川大学出版社
书　　号	ISBN 978-7-5614-7849-3
印前制作	墨创文化
印　　刷	四川盛图彩色印刷有限公司
成品尺寸	100mm×160mm
印　　张	3.25
字　　数	127 千字
版　　次	2020 年 12 月第 1 版
印　　次	2020 年 12 月第 1 次印刷
定　　价	25.00 元

◆ 读者邮购本书，请与本社发行科联系。
电话：(028)85408408/(028)85401670/
(028)86408023　邮政编码：610065

◆ 本社图书如有印装质量问题，请寄回出版社调换。

◆ 网址：http://press.scu.edu.cn

四川大学出版社
微信公众号

《四川大学华西医院实用新冠肺炎汉英词汇速查手册》

编委会

主　审：程南生　曾　勇

主　编：谢　红　廖明恒　卿　平

副主编：郝晓婷　于志渊　黄纪伟　蒋　艳

编　者：（排名不分先后）

冯　梅　廖灯彬　高永莉　李　红　李　玉

彭文涛　游丛毓　王　旭　王　澎　尹俊波

陈玉娟　王浩源　张雅妮　纪鉴芮　陈科润

张天杰　李　雅　苟慎菊　唐思琪　张历涵

毕思伟　葛　格　程扬帆　任硕芳　王　通

陈馨韵　朱昱州　董依廷　姜　亨　余泓彬

汪曼妮　唐泽先　黄　玥　周　健　傅晓莹

王嘉毅　黄静雯　王　煦　杨子涵　熊　婉

林东涛　刁凯悦　高　慧　夏　超　尹　为

郭　文　申永春　蔡俊君　邓丽侠　唐友银

朱星宇　代水平　童　翔　冉启惠　余　淳

陈利平　郭　军　张雨薇　范　红　刘　丹

杨　雪　邱　实　王定玺　李　蓉　华雨薇

文宁远　许　莹　杨　磊

Preface
前言

2020年1月以来，在以习近平同志为核心的党中央的坚强领导下，全国人民齐心协力，广大医务工作者顽强拼搏，同新型冠状病毒肺炎（Corona virus Disease 2019，COVID-19）（以下简称“新冠肺炎”）疫情进行了艰苦卓绝的斗争，取得了举世瞩目的成绩，目前国内疫情防控形势积极向好。然而，随着新冠肺炎疫情在全球快速蔓延，世界卫生组织宣布新冠肺炎疫情已具有大流行特征，形势令人担忧。习近平指出，疫情没有国界，世界各国是休戚与共的命运共同体。在中国抗疫的关键时期，中国得到来自各方的支持，在他国遭遇挑战的困难时刻，中国感同身受，以大国担当的责任和勇气，积极伸出援手，向出现疫情扩散的一些国家提供力所能及的物资援助，派遣抗疫医疗专家万里驰援，分享防控经验，开展药物和疫苗联合研发。只有全球携手合作，才能共克时艰，战胜疫情。

在这种背景下，针对COVID-19的医学国际合作与交流显得格外迫切和重要。但是，新冠肺炎的突然出现令所有的国家、所有的学科、所有的领域措手不及，

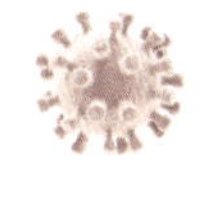

我们需要一本有关新冠肺炎的中英文词句工具书，以扫除跨国医疗援助和合作中的语言障碍。

针对这一问题，四川大学华西临床医学院 / 华西医院迅速启动《四川大学华西医院实用新冠肺炎汉英词汇速查手册》的编撰工作。团队成员主要包括战斗在国内外抗疫战线的华西及兄弟医疗单位医护人员、医学英语师资、国内外华西医学生等，具备良好的专业素质和语言能力。团队成员查阅了大量的新冠肺炎相关医学文献、音频视频等媒体资料以及医疗和护理情景对话专业书籍，抗疫一线医护人员还根据自己的临床经验提供了常用新冠肺炎高频词汇，并亲自编写了多个模拟病例模板。在编写过程中，团队成员夜以继日，对本手册总体结构以及各章节内容进行了多次讨论，反复修订，精益求精，终于在近日完成了本书的编撰工作。

本书内容丰富，学科涵盖面广，贴近临床实践。全书共分为十一个章节，涵盖了新冠肺炎高频词条、病程记录及多科会诊模板、常见疾病诊断、症状及临床体征、病史信息、常用检查检验、胸部影像学检查及诊断、一般及特殊治疗、常用药物及医疗耗材、护理相关、医院感染及医疗流程、常用医学缩略词等内容。

本手册中英文对照，用词和翻译都尽量贴近临床思维和运用习惯，兼顾实用性、针对性、可操作性和详尽性原则。

本书作为一本针对新冠肺炎的中英文速查手册，可以帮助抗疫国际合作扫除语言沟通障碍，也可作为本科医学英语、护理英语和留学生医学中文的教学参考资料。

在本手册即将出版之际，非常感谢院领导及各部门的大力支持！感谢参与编写、审校工作的各位老师和同学们的辛苦付出！

尽管我们参考了大量资料，反复修改并查漏补缺，但是本书仍然可能存在不少错漏之处，敬请批评指正。

谢红

2020 年 8 月

Contents
目录

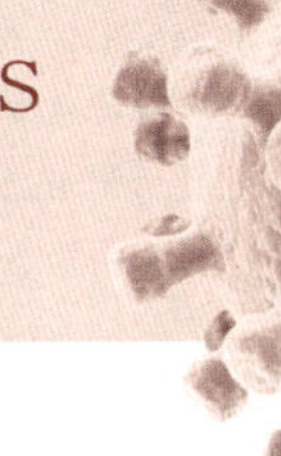

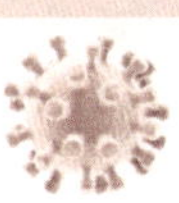

第一章　新冠肺炎高频词条及短句

新冠肺炎常见症状

新型冠状病毒肺炎	Coronavirus disease 2019, COVID-19（WHO 推荐名称）
初始症状	Initial symptom
异常	Abnormality
呼吸困难	Dyspnea
呼吸短促	Shortness of breath
缺氧	Hypoxia
发绀	Cyanosis
咳嗽	Cough
干咳	Dry cough
咳痰	Expectoration / Wet cough
痰液	Sputum
黏液痰	Mucous sputum
脓痰	Purulent sputum
喷嚏	Sneeze
咽痛	Sore throat/Pharyngalgia
发热	Fever
寒战	Shiver
畏寒	Chill
疲劳	Fatigue / Feel tired
头痛	Headache
头晕	Dizziness
食欲不振	Anorexia / Have no appetite

恶心	Nausea / Want to vomit
呕吐	Vomit
腹痛	Abdominal pain / Stomachache
腹泻	Diarrhea
肌痛	Myalgia / Muscle pain
咯血	Hemoptysis
盗汗	Night sweat
潮热	Hot flash

旅行史 / 暴露史 / 流行病学史

曾去过……	Have traveled/been to...
曾接触过……	Have contacted with...
疫区	Affected area
聚餐	Dine together
聚集 / 集会	Gathering
高危患者	High-risk patient
居家令	Stay-at-home policy
自我隔离	Self-isolation/Guarantine

常见慢性基础疾病

合并症	Comorbidity
高血压	Hypertension, HTN
糖尿病	Diabetes mellitus, DM
肿瘤	Tumor
肺癌	Lung cancer
肺结核	Pulmonary tuberculosis

慢性阻塞性肺病	Chronic obstructive pulmonary disease, COPD
慢性肺部疾病	Chronic lung disease
高脂血症	Hyperlipidemia
哮喘	Asthma
免疫缺陷	Immunodeficiency
HIV 感染	HIV infection

常用检查检验

胸部 X 光片	Chest X-Ray, CXR
高分辨率 CT	High-resolution computed tomography, HRCT
胸部 CT	Chest CT
单侧的	Unilateral
双侧的	Bilateral
磨玻璃影	Ground-glass opacification, GGO
胸腔积液	Pleural effusion
标本	Specimen
鼻咽拭子	Nasopharyngeal swab
口咽拭子	Oropharyngeal swab
血常规	Blood routine/Complete blood count
白细胞减少	Leukopenia
淋巴细胞减少	Lymphopenia
动脉血气分析	Arterial blood gas, ABG
动脉血氧分压	Arterial partial pressure of oxygen, PaO_2
二氧化碳分压	Partial pressure of carbon dioxide, $PaCO_2$

血氧饱和度	Oxygen saturation, O_2sat or SaO_2
氧合指数	Oxygenation index, OI
基因组测序	Genome sequencing

常见病原体 / 鉴别诊断

新型冠状病毒	Severe Acute Respiratory Syndrome Coronavirus 2, SARS-CoV-2
冠状病毒	Coronavirus
流行性感冒病毒	Influenza virus
腺病毒	Adenovirus
支原体	Mycoplasma
鲍曼不动杆菌	*Acinetobacter baumannii*, AB
铜绿假单胞菌	*Pseudomonas aeruginosa*, PA
耐甲氧西林金黄色葡萄球菌	Methicillin-resistant Staphylococcus aureus, MRSA
耐万古霉素金黄色葡萄球菌	Vancomycin-resistant Staphylococcus aureus, VRSA
耐万古霉素肠球菌	Vancomycin-resistant enterococcus, VRE
耐碳青霉烯类肺炎克雷伯杆菌	Carbapenem-resistant Klebsiella pneumoniae, CRKP
产气荚膜梭菌	Clostridium perfringen

一般治疗及护理

知情同意书	Informed consent form
普食	Full diet
流质饮食	Liquid diet
半流质饮食	Semi-liquid diet

氧疗	Oxygen therapy
鼻导管	Nasal cannula
面罩氧疗	Mask oxygen therapy
高流量氧疗	High flow oxygen therapy
球囊面罩	Bag valve mask, BVM
无创机械通气	Non-invasive mechanical ventilation
有创机械通气	Invasive mechanical ventilation
呼吸机	Ventilator / Respirator
气管插管	Tracheal intubation
气管切开	Tracheotomy
人工肺 / 体外膜肺氧合	Extracorporeal membrane oxygenation, ECMO
雾化吸入	Aerosol inhalation
吸痰	Sputum suction
祛痰	Dispelling phlegm
稀化黏液	Loosen mucus
肺复张	Lung recruitment
卧床休息	Bed rest
俯卧位	Prone position / Lie on the stomach
抬高床头（尾）	Raise the head (foot) of the bed
预防压力性损伤	Prevent pressure ulcer
压力性损伤	Pressure ulcer Bedsore
留置导尿	Reserved urethral catheter / Indwelling catheterization
导尿管	Forley catheter
冷（热）敷	Apply an ice or a warm pack

常用药物

α－干扰素	α-interferon
瑞德西韦	Remdesivir
洛匹那韦	Lopinavir
利托那韦	Ritonavir
利巴韦林	Ribavirin
磷酸氯喹	Chloroquine phosphate
去甲肾上腺素	Norepinephrine
低分子肝素	Low-molecular-weight heparin, LMWH
甲泼尼龙	Methylprednisolone
呋塞米	Furosemide

重症治疗常用词汇

急性呼吸窘迫综合征	Acute respiratory distress syndrome, ARDS
低氧血症	Hypoxemia
呼吸衰竭	Respiratory failure
脓毒性休克	Septic shock
代谢性酸中毒	Metabolic acidosis
出凝血功能障碍	Coagulopathy
弥漫性血管内凝血	Disseminated intravascular coagulation, DIC
多器官功能衰竭	Multiple organ failure, MOF
急性心脏损伤	Acute cardiac injury
心律失常	Arrhythmia
肝功能异常	Liver dysfunction
急性肾损伤	Acute kidney injury, AKI

继发细菌感染	Secondary bacterial infection
连续性肾脏替代治疗	Continuous renal replacement therapy, CRRT
皮疹	Rash
心肺复苏	Cardiopulmonary resuscitation, CPR

院感及个人防护

针刺伤	Needle stick injury
一次性	Disposable
穿	Don/ Put on
脱	Doff / Take off
穿脱隔离衣	Donning and Doffing isolation gown
二级防护	Level II protection
个人防护用品	Personal protective equipment, PPE
洗手衣	Scrub
工作帽	Head cover / Surgical cap
医用防护口罩	Medical protective mask
外科口罩	Surgical mask
产生气溶胶的操作	Aerosol-generating procedures, AGPs
N95 口罩	N95 mask
半罩式防护呼吸器	Elastomeric half-mask respirator
动力空气净化呼吸器	Powered air purifying respirator, PAPR
眼部防护	Eye protection
护目镜	Goggles / Safety glasses
面屏	Face shield
医用防护服	Medical protective gown

一次性隔离衣	Disposable gown
乳胶手套	Latex gloves
靴套	Boot cover
避污纸	Paper towel
医院感染预防与控制	Nosocomial infection prevention and control
清洁区	Clean area
潜在污染区	Potentially contaminated area
缓冲区	Buffer area / Doffing area
污染区	Contaminated area
负压病房	Negative pressure ward
丢弃	Dispose
负压担架	Negative pressure stretcher
锐器伤	Sharp injuries

常用短句 / 短语

新型冠状病毒阳性
SARS-CoV-2 positive
间隔 24 小时以上 2 次新型冠状病毒阴性
The second swab test of SARS-CoV-2 is negative more than 24 hours apart. Two consecutive negative tests for SARS-CoV-2 at least 24 hours apart between swabs.
有……症状
Has symptoms of ... Have an attack of ... Presence of ... Present with ...

没有……症状
Absence of ... No [+ 症状]
伴有……
Be accompanied by...
与……有关
Be associated with...
HCV 抗体阳性
HCV antibody positive
流感检测阴性
Flu swab was negative.
在正常范围内
Within the normal range
（采血管）颠倒混匀 5 ～ 8 次
Gently mix the blood collection tube by inverting 5–8 times
胸腔积液培养无异常
No abnormality in pleural effusion culture
痰涂片查见结核分枝杆菌。
Sputum smear shows MTB (*M. tuberculosis*).
胸腔积液涂片查见结核分枝杆菌、真菌、细菌。
Pleural effusion smear shows MTB, fungi and bacteria.
尿常规提示脓细胞++。
Urinalysis suggests pus cells ++ .
血培养提示耐甲氧西林金黄色葡萄球菌。
Blood culture detects MRSA.

不排除泛耐药鲍曼不动杆菌感染可能
Cannot exclude PDRAB (pan-drug resistant *A. Baumannii*) infections
肺部合并真菌感染
Pulmonary fungal infection
混合性感染
Mixed infection
多发磨玻璃小斑片影
Multiple patchy shadow-like GGO
CT 见双肺多发斑片影伴有空洞
Bilateral multiple patchy shadows and cavities seen on CT
右侧胸腔积液（最深 4 厘米）
Right pleural effusion (maximum depth of 4 cm)
胸腔引流 1 200 毫升淡黄色清亮积液
Chest drainage of 1, 200 mL of clear yellow effusion

第二章　实用英文病历模板

病历文书相关词汇

病历文书	Medical records
入院记录	Admission note
主诉	Chief complaint, CC
现病史	History of present illness, HPI
流行病学史	History of travel, occupation, contact and cluster, TOCC
既往史	Past medical history , PMH
个人史	Personal history, PH
家庭史	Family history, FHx
体格检查	Physical examination, PE
瞳孔等大等圆，对光反射灵敏	Pupils equally round, and reactive to light, PERRL
病史汇报	Briefing
无特殊	Non-contributory / Unremarkable
病程记录	Progress note
查房	Round
主治医师查房	Senior round
教授 / 全科查房	Grand round
转科记录	Transfer note
出院记录	Discharge note

入院病历提纲

主诉 （Chief complaint）
Coughing and shortness of breath［症状］for 2 weeks［时间］

现病史 （History of present illness ）
The patient started cough, chest tightness［ 症状 ］since 2 weeks［ 时 间 ］ago. It is associated with yellow sputum, sore throat and muscle weakness［ 伴随症状 ］, no/without fever or diarrhea［ 阴性症状 ］. He cannot even stand up［ 影响功能到什么程度 ］.
A few days after his symptom appear, he visited XXX hospital. Throat swab test was SARS-CoV-2 positive. The CT scan was unremarkable.［ 辅查阳性写前面，阴性写后面 ］He received antibiotic treatment［ 治 疗 方 案 ］. His shortness of breath became severe［ 治疗转归 ］. His family member brought him to the hospital.
既往史及个人史（Past medical history and personal history）
Hypertension was stably controlled by Nifedipine extended-release tablets［ 药物 ］.
Smoking 1 pack per day for 20 years［ 剂量 + 时间 ］, no drinking / alcohol abuse.
家庭史（Family history）
Family history was unremarkable.
Family history of Type 2 Diabetes, mother, sister and aunt［ 疾病，亲属 ］.
流行病学史（History of travel, occupation, contact and cluster）
He travelled to［+ 地点 ］.
He worked in［+ 工作地点 ］.
Two clients were diagnosed as COVID-19［ 环境接触 ］.
He contacted his friend on March 20th, who was diagnosed as COVID-19 yesterday［ 密切接触 ］.
社会史（Social history）
Truck driver［ 职业 ］
Home with wife, 2 kids

体格检查（Physical examination）
意识：Alert/normal/tired looking/sleepy looking/comatose
体征：T 36.3℃, P 90 bpm, R 20 breaths/min, BP 151/65 mmHg, SaO_2 98% (FiO_2 21%)
查体：Coorperative / uncoorperative
瞳孔等大等圆，对光反射灵敏：PERRL, L 2 mm, R 3 mm
对光反射迟钝：Sluggish reactive to light
瞳孔扩大固定：Pupils dilated, no reactive to light
瞳孔针尖样：Pin-pointed pupil
无法查体：PE unperformable
辅助检查（Investigation）
SARS-CoV-2 positive in throat swab
目前诊断（Diagnosis）
COVID-19 Hypertension
诊疗计划（Plan）
氧疗：Nasal catheter 2 L/min; oxygen mask 10 L/min; non-rebreather mask［储氧面罩］
无创呼吸机：Noninvasive ventilation Bipap/CPAP［+ 各种参数］
机械通气：Endotracheal tube/ Tracheotomy tube with A/C, SIMV［+ 各种模式］
常规：Cardiac monitoring, Blood sugar monitoring q4h/q12h［见治疗］
检查：Investigation［+ 检查项目］
治疗：treatment［+ 药物名称 + 剂量 + 用法 + 频次］
沟通：Explain diagnosis, treatment plan and prognosis to patient/relatives

病史汇报示例

病例一

女性，73岁，“发热、腹泻12天”，无明显诱因出现发热，体温最高38.9℃，伴轻度腹泻、背痛，无乏力、呼吸困难等，家中自查血氧饱和度89%，已口服阿比多尔3天。

既往“高血压”，近日血压160/90 mmHg，停药1周。有“焦虑性抑郁症”，平素服用盐酸曲唑酮片、酒石酸唑吡坦片治疗，对青霉素过敏，表现皮疹、眩晕。

Case 1

This is a 73-year-old female presenting with fever and diarrhea for 12 days. Pt developed fever with no identifiable cause, highest temperature thirty-eight point nine degrees Celsius, associated with mild diarrhea, back pain. Pt denies fatigue and dyspnea. Oxygen saturation at home was 89 percent. She has been taking Arbidol (Umifenovir) for 3 days.

Past medical history is significant for hypertension, recent blood pressure is 160 over 90 millimeters of mercury, off anti-hypertensives for one week. She has mixed anxiety-depression, on trazodone hydrochloride tablets and zolpidem tartrate tablets.

Allergic to penicillin, reactions were rash and dizziness.

病例二

男性，67 岁，“咳嗽、咳痰 30 天，呼吸困难 2 天”入院。患者反复高热，体温最高 39.8℃。社区医院考虑“重症肺炎（细菌、病毒感染），I 型呼吸衰竭，低白蛋白血症，重度营养不良，肝功能不全，类风湿性关节炎”。昨夜送至我院急诊，肺泡灌洗液行新型冠状病毒 RNA 核酸检测回示“阳性”，痰液新型冠状病毒 RNA 核酸阴性。既往史、个人史无特殊。

Case 2

This is a 67-year-old male presenting with productive cough for 30 days and dyspnea for 2 days. Pt has recurrent high fever, highest temperature 39.8 degrees Celsius. The community hospital suspected severe pneumonia (bacterial, viral infection), hypoxemic respiratory failure, hypoalbuminemia, severe malnutrition, liver dysfunction, rheumatoid arthritis. Last night, patient was sent to our ER. The SARS-CoV-2 PCR is positive from bronchoalveolar lavage(BAL), negative in sputum sample. Non-contributory past medical history and personal history.

病程记录提纲

病程记录 Progress note / Round note / Grand round note
Level of consciousness, LOC Alert/conscious/tired looking/sleepy looking/comatose Present illness T 36.3℃ , P 90 bpm, R 20 breaths/min, BP 151/65 mmHg, SaO_2 98% (FiO_2 40%) Dehydrated/Well hydrated [+ 症状或体征， 见下] Investigation [+ 检查名称] Treatment plan [+ 药物名称 + 剂量 + 用法 + 频次]

会诊记录提纲

会诊记录
Consultation note
[记录别人的会诊意见]
XXX department consulted: diagnosis: XXXXX.
suggestion: XXXX.

核心用语

意识清晰程度
Level of consciousness, LOC

清醒 / 嗜睡 / 烦躁 / 谵妄 / 昏睡 / 昏迷
Conscious/ Somnolent / Dysphoria / Delirious / Stuporous / Comatose
精神欠佳
Tired looking/Sleepy looking
一般情况：好 / 一般 / 略差 / 差
General condition: Very good / Good / Fair / Poor
生命体征平稳
Vital signs are stable.
病危，生命体征平稳
Critically ill but stable
明显较前好转
Feel much better
（患者的）精神、食欲、睡眠、活动较前好转 / 无变化
Patient's spirits, appetite, sleep and activity have improved / not changed.
患者神志清楚，反复要求下床，多次劝说无效。
The patient was conscious and ambulated despite of dissuasion.
患者治疗配合度差
The patient had poor compliance.
患者气管插管，镇静状态，呼吸机模式 A/C
Patient sedated, in Assist/Control mode ventilation
意识清醒，呼吸机辅助呼吸
Conscious, on mechanical ventilation

呼吸机无异常事件发生
Ventilator works fine./No ventilator-associated events
血氧饱和度维持在 98% 左右
SaO_2 around 98%
今晨体温 38℃ / 100℉
This morning T 38℃ / 100℉
反复发热
Recurrent fever
无发热、畏寒及盗汗
No fever, chill or night sweat
咳嗽、咳黄色痰伴血丝
Coughing, producing yellow, blood-tinged sputum
咳白色泡沫痰
Coughing up frothy sputum
胸闷、呼吸短促较前加重
Worsening chest distress and shortness of breath
双肺叩诊呈浊音
Dullness on percussion in both Lungs
双肺呼吸增粗
Coarse breath sounds in both Lungs
双下肺可闻及少许中细湿啰音
Fine / medium crackles in bilateral lower lung lobes
双下肺呼吸音稍低
Diminished breath sounds in both lower lung lobes
营养状况差
Poor nutrition

24 小时液体平衡情况：总入量 2 450 毫升，总出量 3 300 毫升
24h fluid balance situation: total input 2, 450 mL, output 3, 300 mL
胸腔引流 1 200 毫升淡黄色清亮胸水
Chest drained 1, 200 mL of clear yellow pleural fluid.
治疗计划
Treatment plan
继续目前治疗，观察病情变化。
Continue current treatment, and observe patients.
复查提示低白蛋白血症，今日予以静滴人血白蛋白20克纠正。
Re-examination revealed hypoalbuminemia, human albumin 20 g iv planned.
密切观察患者心功能，警惕暴发性病毒性心肌病。
Given the concern of fulminant viral cardiomyopathy, careful observation of the patient's heart function is required.
今日复查新型冠状病毒核酸检测（咽拭子 + 肛拭子）。
Repeat throat and anal swab tests for SARS-CoV-2 today.
病情稳定，可以转普通病房治疗。
The patient is stable and can be transferred to the general ward.

病程记录示例

病例一

A 先生神志清楚，胸闷、呼吸短促较前有所改善，无发热、鼻塞、流涕、咽痛等症状，24 小时静脉入量 1 600 毫升，饮食 160 毫升，小便 1 000 毫升，大便未解。

患者口服克力芝第三天，未出现恶心、呕吐等反应，今日调整剂量为 500 毫克，每日两次。安排明日复查 T 淋巴细胞，后日复查胸部 CT。治疗上停止鼻导管吸氧，停用布地奈德、特布他林雾化吸入，余治疗同原计划，密切观察患者病情变化。

Case 1

Mr. A was conscious, his chest distress and shortness of breath were relieved, and he had no fever, stuffy nose, runny nose, or sore throat and so on. Over the past 24 hours, 1, 600 mL of fluid was administered iv, 160 mL was consumed orally and urine output was 1, 000 mL. No poop.

This is the 3rd day of oral Kaletra (lopinavir/ritonavir). He complains of no adverse events, such as nausea or vomiting. Plan to adjust dose to 500 mg po bid today. Other plans include repeating T lymphocyte counts test tomorrow and chest CT scan the day after tomorrow. Discontinue nasal cannula of oxygen, the aerosol inhalation of budesonide and terbutaline. Continue other symptomatic treatment. Observe the patient closely.

病例二

今日 16:00 查看 B 先生神志清楚，精神尚可，呼吸平稳，鼻导管吸氧 3 升 / 分钟；8 小时静脉入 0 毫升，食入 1 070 毫升，小便 680 毫升，大便 0 次。

查体：T 36.3℃，P 79 次 / 分，R 19 次 / 分，BP 127/61 mmHg，SaO_2 97%（FiO_2 40%）。双侧瞳孔等大等圆，直径约 2 毫米，光反射灵敏。口唇无发绀，双肺叩诊呈清音；胸部、心脏、腹部听诊不能完成，双下肢不肿。辅助检查：［动脉血气分析］氧合指数 193。

下一步计划：患者 3 日内无发热，安排复查新型冠状病毒核酸（咽拭子 + 肛拭子）；复查胸部 CT，继续完善床旁心电图及双下肢静脉血管彩超；予以静滴人血白蛋白 10 克纠正低白蛋白血症，加用布地奈德 + 特布他林雾化，继续抗病毒及对症治疗，密切观察患者病情变化。

Case 2

16:00 progress note:

Mr. B was conscious, overall status improved. Inhale O_2 3 L/min with nasal cannula. 8-hour input: 0 mL iv, 1, 070 mL oral with food, 680 ml urine. No poop.

PE: T 36.3℃ , P 79 bpm, R 19 breaths/min, BP 127/61 mmHg, SaO_2 97% (FiO_2 40%). PERRL, about 2 mm. No cyanosis on the lips. Both lungs percussion showed resonant sound. Auscultation of chest, heart, and abdomen were not achieved. No pitting edema in the legs. Investigations: ABG, OI=193.

Treatment and plan: If Mr. B did not have fever within 3 days, he can take another SARS-CoV-2 PCR test (throat swab + anal swab), and chest CT test. Continue to improve bedside EKG and DVT screening color ultrasound of both lower extremities. Required correction of hypoalbuminemia, human albumin 10 g iv and, the aerosol inhalation of budesonide, terbutaline inhalation. Antiviral and symptomatic treatment will be continued. Observe the patient closely.

病例三

晨 8 点查房：

T 36.8℃，P 80 次 / 分，R 20 次 / 分，BP 112/62 mmHg，SaO_2 93%（FiO_2 41%），C 先生神志清楚，查体合作；呼吸稍快，口唇无发绀，双肺叩诊呈清音，胸部、心脏、腹部听诊不能完成，双下肢不肿。补充辅助检查：[动脉血气分析] 氧合指数 160。[血常规] [血浆乳酸] [血生化] [血脂] [电解质] [凝血功能] [输血前全套] [淋巴细胞亚群测定] [T 细胞计数] [炎性因子] [真菌 G 试验] [BNP] [心肌标志物] 未见异常。[流感病毒核酸检测] 阴性，[TORCH] 阴性。

下一步计划：患者血常规提示淋巴细胞数量进行性减少，通过鼻咽拭子检测新型冠状病毒核酸，结果阳性，流感病毒筛查阴性，血气分析提示 I 型呼吸衰竭，经普通吸氧，氧合指数低于 100，目前病危，予以高流量吸氧，继续监测生命体征、血糖，治疗上已给予干扰素雾化抗病毒；血钠及血钾低，予以补充电解质。今日专家组讨论后加用克立芝 250 毫克，每日两次，进行抗病毒治疗。明日继续复查血常规、血生化、电解质、胸部 CT。患者有气管插管操作可能，予以单间负压病房隔离，医务人员进入病房时进行二级防护，气道操作时给予正压头罩防护。通过电话向患者及家属交代病情，并获得理解。

Case 3

8:00 a.m. progress note:

PE: T 36.8°C, P 80 bpm, R 20 breaths/min, BP 112/62 mmHg, SaO_2 93% (FiO_2 41%).

Mr. C was conscious and cooperative. A slight tachypnea was noted. No cyanosis on the lips. Pulmonary percussion showed resonant sound. Thoracic, cardiac, and abdominal auscultation could not be achieved. No pitting edema in the legs. ABG revealed OI=160. The results of [+different tests] were unremarkable. The patient was negative for rapid flu test and TORCH test.

Treatment and plan:

Mr. C's lymphocytes decreased progressively from latest CBC. His nasopharyngeal swab was positive for SARS-CoV-2 and negative for influenza virus. ABG revealed type I respiratory failure with OI<100 on NC oxygen. Given the critical condition, high-flow oxygen was prescribed with continuous monitoring of vital signs and blood glucose. Nebulized interferon was initiated. Hyponatremia and hypokalemia were noticed and electrolyte was replaced. Consulting experts suggested a complemented antiviral therapy of Kaletra (lopinavir/ritonavir) 250 mg bid today. Continue monitoring CBC, blood biochemistry, electrolyte panels and repeat chest CT test in the next day.

As intubation & extubation should occur in a negative pressure room, Mr. C has been currently moved to an isolated negative pressure ward. Level II protection was required for all healthcare providers. Powered air purifying system was used in aerosol-generating procedures (AGPs) such as intubation. Communication with the patient and his family were achieved over the phone and consent was obtained.

其他文书示例

深静脉置管记录 Central venous catheter (CVC) insertion note

与患者家属沟通并征得同意后，将患者置于去枕仰卧位。采用 Seldinger 技术和无菌操作，在右锁骨中点以下 1 厘米处植入中心静脉导管。导管深度达到 13 厘米后，缝合固定，消毒后用无菌纱布覆盖。胸片显示右肺部未见明显改变。

Communicated with the patient's family and consent was obtained. The patient is placed into a low supine position. CVC inserted at 1 cm below the midpoint of the right clavicle, using Seldinger technique and aseptic technique. The catheter depth is 13 cm, fixed with suture, covered with sterile gauze after disinfection. Chest X-Ray showed no obvious change in right lung.

抢救记录 - 紧急气管插管 Rescue note – Emergency tracheal intubation

气管插管操作记录

日期：<___>

时间：〈___〉

插管指征：呼吸窘迫

住院医师：〈___〉

主治医师：〈___〉

操作前核对患者、操作过程、定位、体位和特殊设备（如果适用的话）。取平卧位，使用镇静剂 XX 毫克与肌松剂 XX 毫克。使用球囊通气。在口咽部插入 MAC T3 喉镜片及可视喉镜，此时获得声带部 1 级视野（即充分暴露声门）。插入 7.5 号气管导管并在可视化喉镜下通过声带，然后移除管芯。在 CO_2 检测仪中可观察到正常的 CO_2 波形（未用可删去）。因着防护服未能完成听诊双侧呼吸音。气管导管放置在距离门齿 23 厘米处。整个操作过程都在主治医生指导下完成。

进行胸部 X 光检查以排除气胸和确认气管插管位置。

操作总时长：〈___〉

患者耐受性良好，无并发症发生。

Endotracheal Intubation Procedure Note

Date: <_____>

Time: <_____>

Indication: Respiratory Distress

Resident: <_____>

Attending: <_____>

A time-out was completed verifying correct patient, procedure, site, positioning, and special equipment if applicable. The patient was placed in a supine position. Sedation was obtained using <sedative XX mg>, and additionally with <muscle relaxants XX mg>. The patient was ventilated using an Ambu bag. The MAC T3 blade / glidescope was used and inserted into the oropharynx at which time there was a grade 1 view of the vocal cords. A 7.5-french endotracheal tube was inserted and visualized going through the vocal cords. The stylet was removed. Colorimetric change was visualized on the CO_2 meter Breath sounds cannot be heard because of barrier gown. The endotracheal tube was placed at 23 cm < 深 度 >, measured at the incisor. Attending was present for the entire procedure.

A chest X-ray was ordered to assess for pneumothorax and verify endotracheal tube placement.

Estimated time used for the procedure: <____>

The patient tolerated the procedure well and there were no complications.

腰椎穿刺记录 Lumbar puncture note

与患者家属沟通并征得同意后，患者取右侧卧位，双手抱膝，尽量弯曲脊柱。采用 9 号针，在无菌环境下进行。取清亮脑脊液 15 毫升送检，具体检查包括细胞计数、生化检查、细菌培养、耐药性、真菌培养等。

Communicated with the patient's family and obtained consent. The patient is placed in the right side, holding the knees with both hands and curling as much as possible. Lumbar puncture was done under aseptic technique using 9# needle. Clear CSF 15 mL was sent for investigations: cell count, biochemical test, bacterial culture, drug resistance, fungal culture, etc.

抢救记录（病例一）Rescue note（Case 1）

A 先生烦躁不安，胡言乱语，拒绝使用无创呼吸机，拒绝吸氧，反复劝说无效，呼吸频率 30 次 / 分左右，脉搏血氧饱和度 70% 左右，口唇及甲床发绀，血气分析示患者 I 型呼吸衰竭，病情危重，组织抢救。患者目前右美托咪定静脉泵入，加用丙泊酚加强镇静，并给予盐酸瑞芬太尼对症处理，待患者安静下继续给予无创呼吸机支持呼吸（吸气气道正压 10 cmH2O，呼气气道正压 6 cmH2O），人机配合尚可，呼吸较前平稳，吸氧浓度由 100% 逐渐下调至 65%，脉搏血氧饱和度维持在 97% 左右，心率在 90 次 / 分左右，血压 123/81 mmHg，抢救成功。

Mr. A developed delirium, refused to use the noninvasive ventilator, refused to take oxygen, repeated persuasion could not help him calm down. Respiratory rate increased to about 30 breaths/min, SaO_2 dropped to about 70%, cyanosis was noticed. ABG showed the patient had type I respiratory failure, situation was critical. Rescue was performed The dexmedetomidine infusion was continued throughout the iv pump, added propofol and remifentanil iv for acceptable sedation. Mr. A was given non-invasive ventilator support for breathing (IPAP 10 cmH2O, EPAP 6 cmH2O). After treatment, patient's ventilation improved, FiO_2 gradually reduced from 100% to 65%, SaO_2 was maintained at about 97%, the heart rate returned to about 90 bpm, and the BP was 123/81 mmHg. ROSC.

抢救记录（病例二）Rescue note（Case 2）

12:20 B 小姐出现咳痰费力，呼吸困难，喘息，可见三凹征，心率最快增至 190 次 / 分，呼吸达 35 次 / 分左右，给予吸痰，吸出较多脓痰及血性痰液，并有血痂，并予以多索茶碱及甲泼尼龙静脉输入、特布他林及布地奈德雾化吸入解痉平喘，胺碘酮控制心室率等对症处理，无创呼吸机氧气浓度上调至 100%，但 SaO_2 最高波动于 85%~88%。完善气管插管前准备，镇静镇痛后于 14:15 给予气管插管，使用 7.0 号气管导管，插管深度自门齿 20 厘米，连接氧气检测仪，检查插管在位，妥善固定。插管后有创呼吸机容控通气，继续予以咪达唑仑镇静及瑞芬太尼镇痛，插管后复测血压 63/37 mmHg，予以多巴胺静脉泵入升压治疗。治疗后患者血压在 100/60 mmHg，根据患者氧合逐步下调吸氧浓度至 50%，14:40 患者心率 112 次 / 分，呼吸 21 次 / 分，血压 119/65 mmHg，SaO_2 98%，抢救成功。

At 12:20, Ms. B developed difficulty expectoration, dyspnea, wheezing with chest retractions. The heart rate increased to 190 bpm, and the respiratory rate reached about 35 breaths/min. She was given suction, and much purulent and bloody sputum were extracted, as well as clots. The patient was given doxofylline iv and methylprednisolone iv, terbutaline and budesonide inhalation to relieve spasm and improve ventilation, amiodarone to control ventricular rate, and other symptomatic treatment. FiO_2 of noninvasive ventilator was raised to 100%, but the maximum SaO_2 fluctuated between 85%-88%, decided intubation. At 14:15, after sedation and analgesia, Ms. B was given tracheal intubation with a 7.0 mm internal diameter standard endotracheal tube. The tube was secured with its 20 cm mark at the incisor, connected O_2 detector to verify position and properly fixed. Started the patient on a volume-controlled ventilation, and continued to give midazolam for sedation and remifentanil for analgesia. Re-measured BP was 63/37 mmHg after intubation. Dopamine was given by intravenous pumping to elevate blood pressure. After treatment, the patient's BP was 100/60 mmHg, and the FiO_2 was gradually reduced to 50% based on oxygenation. At 14:40, the patient's heart rate was 112 bpm, the respiratory rate was 21 breaths/min, BP was 119/65 mmHg, SaO_2 was 98%.ROSC.

交班汇报 - 普通病区 Shift exchange in general ward

病区原有患者 80 例，转入 ICU 3 例，收入院 40 例。

CPR 0 例，气管插管 1 例，无创机械通气 1 例，有创机械通气 9 例。1 例出院，无死亡病例。目前，共有 83 例患者，其中 12 例正在 ICU 接受治疗。

新报告多重耐药细菌感染（VRSA）1 例。

本病区目前有 1 例胸痛患者正在接受治疗。

There were 80 patients initially on our shift. We moved 3 patients to the ICU and 40 to the inpatient wards.

There were 0 CPR, 1 tracheal intubation, 1 noninvasive mechanical ventilation, 9 invasive mechanical ventilations on the ground. There were 1 discharge and 0 death. Up to now, we have 83 patients and 12 of them are under treatment in ICU.

One patient was reported multiple drug resistant bacteria infection (VRSA).

There is 1 patient with chest pain currently receiving treatment in our area.

转科记录 Transferred note

入院后予以心电监护，面罩吸氧 5 升 / 分，气垫床预防压疮，间歇式压力充气泵预防深静脉血栓。患者胸闷、呼吸短促症状呈进行性加重，血气分析提示患者氧合指数低于 200，予以高流量吸氧（流量 35 升 / 分、氧浓度 45%），并予以干扰素雾化抗病毒，静脉注射乙酰半胱氨酸改善肺间质纤维化，人血白蛋白维持血浆渗透压，及常规对症支持治疗。监护治疗 3 日后患者病情好转，换鼻导管吸氧 5 升 / 分后昨日已停止氧疗，今日转出重症监护病房。

After admission, the patient was on continuous cardiac monitoring, and received oxygen inhale 5 L/min with mask. Applied air bed to prevent pressure ulcers, intermittent pneumatic compression (IPC) devices to prevent deep vein thrombosis. The patient's chest tightness and shortness of breath exacerbated, ABG revealed an oxygenation index lower than 200. The patient was given high-flow oxygen at a rate of 35 L/min (FiO_2 45%), interferon nebulization, acetylcysteine intravenous infusion, human albumin and symptomatic treatment. After 3 days of intensive treatment, the patient's clinical condition had been improved. Nasal cannula of oxygen (3 L/min) was applied and was discontinued yesterday. The patient was transferred out of the intensive care unit today.

出院记录 Discharge note

女性，50 岁，“间断咳嗽、乏力、发热 1 周，胸痛 1- 天”入院，自述超市购物接触疑似患者，居家观察期间出现咳嗽、乏力等不适，自感发热（体温 37.2℃），2 月 2 日新型冠状病毒 RNA 核酸检测鼻咽拭子阳性，继续居家观察。2 月 8 日无明显诱因出现胸痛不适，呈心前区闷胀痛，心电图提示不排除前间壁心肌梗死可能，收治入院；患者既往“冠心病”，未行治疗。入院后患者复查 [+ 项目] 未见异常，给予吸氧、[其他治疗] 及口服中药治疗后，患者症状好转，间隔 24 小时复查两次核酸检测阴性，符合出院标准。

This is a 50-year-old female, presenting with intermittent cough, fatigue, fever for one week and chest pain for less than one day. She reported contact with a suspected case at the supermarket. During observation period, she developed cough, fatigue, subjective fever (T 37℃). On Feb. 2nd, her SARS-CoV-2 nasopharyngeal swab reported positive, and continued home observation. On Feb. 8th, the patient developed chest pain without any obvious trigger, described it as precordial pain. EKG cannot rule out anteroseptal infarction. PMH is significant for untreated coronary heart disease. The patient was subsequently admitted, had [+different tests], and no abnormalities were found. After giving oxygen and oral Chinese medicine, the patient's symptoms improved. The second swab test of SARS-CoV-2 was negative more than 24 hours apart. Meeting discharge criteria.

会诊记录示例

病例一

病史敬悉，患者老年男性，高血压、糖尿病、痛风病基础，此次因“发热伴乏力、咳嗽”入院。

目前考虑诊断：1. 发热待诊：肺部感染，其他待排？2. 痛风。3. 高血压病。4. Ⅱ型糖尿病？

建议：

1. 患者体温高峰下降，继续莫西沙星抗感染，其余予以化痰等对症处理；

2. 发热时抽培养：完善血沉，CRP，PCT，完善痰涂片（细菌+真菌+分枝杆菌）+痰培养，PPD 皮试，IGRA，TORCH-IgM，呼吸道 13 项病毒、流感抗原筛查，EBV-DNA，CMV-DNA。

3. 请呼吸科、血液内科协助诊治，我科随访。

Case 1

Present & PMH:

The patient was an elderly male with hypertension, diabetes and gout. He was admitted to the hospital due to fever, fatigue and cough.

Diagnoses:

1. FUO: pulmonary infection or others?
2. Gout.
3. Hypertension.
4. Type II diabetes? (to be confirmed) .

Suggestions:

1. Given that the patient's highest temperature has decreased, continue moxifloxacin treatment and symptomatic treatment. Clear sputum symptomatically.

2. Complete ESR, CRP, PCT blood tests, sputum smears (bacteria + fungi + mycobacteria), sputum culture, PPD skin test, IGRA, TORCH-IgM, 13 respiratory viruses screening, influenza antigen screening, EBV-DNA, CMV-DNA, etc. during fever.

3. Consult Respiratory Department, Hematology for advice on diagnosis and treatment. Will follow up.

病例二（呼吸科会诊记录）

诊断：发热待诊。

建议：

1. 血象见中幼粒细胞及晚幼粒细胞，血液系统疾病待排，请血液科会诊；

2. 针对肺部病灶，可继续莫西沙星抗感染，沐舒坦祛痰，泰诺每 8 小时 1 片对症；

3. 患者新型冠状病毒及甲型流感病毒、乙型流感病毒阴性，完善其他病毒检测（呼吸道 13 种病毒、TORCH、EBV-DNA、CMV-DNA）、PCT、痰（痰培养、痰抗酸涂片）、PPD 皮试及 TB-IGRA，必要时血培养。

Case 2

Diagnose: FUO.

Suggestions:

1. Routine CBC count reported elevated myelocyte and metamyelocyte. Hematological diseases to be excluded. Recommend Hematology consultation.

2. For lung lesions, continue antibiotics treatment with moxifloxacin and remove sputum with mucosolvan, add tylenol cold 1-tab prn (q8h at most).

3. The patient was SARS-CoV-2-negative and H1N1-negative. Should perform other viral tests (13 respiratory viruses screening, TORCH, EBV-DNA, CMV-DNA), and serum PCT, sputum tests (sputum culture, sputum antacid smear), PPD skin test and TB-IGRA, blood culture if necessary.

病例三（多科会诊记录）

患者前期影像学提示双肺及胸膜多发结节、多浆膜腔积液。结核？肿瘤？患者现反复低热，贵科已安排相关检查明确病变性质，建议尽可能彩超引导下腹穿，完善腹水脱落细胞、常规、生化、培养及结核相关检查；必要时行 PET-CT、全身骨显象。

Case 3（Multidisciplinary consultation）

The latest chest CT scan showed multiple nodules and pleural, peritoneal and pericardial effusions. Current diagnosis suggests tuberculosis, and differential diagnosis including tumor or others. The patient has repeatedly low fever. Investigation is still pending. It is recommended to arrange color ultrasound-guided abdominal paracentesis, sending peritoneal fluid sample for ascitic fluid cytology, routine, biochemistry, culture and tuberculosis tests. PET-CT and bone SPECT are recommended if necessary.

常见临床医技科室名称

发热门诊	Fever Clinic
急诊科	Emergency Department, ED
感染科	Dept. of Infectious Diseases, ID
心脏内科	Dept. of Cardiology
内分泌科	Dept. of Endocrinology
肾脏内科	Dept. of Nephrology
呼吸内科	Dept. of Respiratory Medicine
胃肠内科	Dept. of Gastroenterology
神经内科	Dept. of Neurology
妇科	Dept. of Gynecology
产科	Dept. of Obstetrics
骨科	Dept. of Orthopedics
胸外科	Dept. of Thoracic Surgery
心脏大血管外科	Dept. of Cardiovascular Surgery
肝胆胰外科	Dept. of Hepato-pancreato-biliary Surgery
胃肠外科	Dept. of Gastrointestinal Surgery
泌尿外科	Dept. of Urology
神经外科	Dept. of Neurosurgery
血管外科	Dept. of Vascular Surgery
移植中心	Transplant Center
临床营养科	Dept. of Nutrition
精神心理科	Dept. of Mental Health
影像介入科	Dept. of Interventional Radiology
心导管室	Cardiac Catheterization Room
消化内镜室	Digestive Endoscopic Center

肿瘤科	Dept. of Oncology
康复科	Dept. of Rehabilitation
皮肤科	Dept. of Dermatology
放疗科	Dept. of Radiotherapy
核医学科	Dept. of Nuclear Medicine
影像科	Dept. of Radiology
超声科	Dept. of Ultrasound
重症监护室	Intensive Care Unit, ICU
麻醉科	Dept. of Anesthesiology
手术室	Operating Room, OR
药剂科	Dept. of Pharmacy
检验科	Dept. of Clinical Laboratory Medicine
院感部门	Dept. of Nosocomial Infection Prevention and Control
隔离病房	Isolation Ward
战地医院	Field Hospital
移动手术间	Mobile Operating Room

现病史

起病情况
无诱因下
with no triggering factors
有……接触史
has close contact with...
有……症状
has symptoms of...
与……有关
be associated with...
伴有……
be accompanied by...
急性……
acute……
慢性……
chronic……
暴发性发病。
The onset was fulminating.
骤起……/ 突然起病伴……
an acute / rapid onset of...accompanied by...
突发突止。
Attacks began and ended abruptly.
因……而突然起病
The attack was precipitated by...

很快发生……
...occurred rapidly
逐渐出现……
gradual onset of...
偶而
occasionally
反复……
recurrent...
一过性发作
transient attack
连续
consistent
时重时轻 / 时好时坏
come and go
发作性……
paroxysmal...
频繁……
frequently...
持续性……
persistent...
间歇性……
intermittent...
频发……
frequent episodes of...
持续不变
remain the same

症状变化
症状好转
improve / be better / make favorable progress
症状减轻
alleviate / relieve / reduce / diminish / ease
症状消失
disappear / vanish / clear up
症状加重
aggravate / exacerbate / be worse / worsen / become heavier
无变化
remain the same / have not changed / have had no changes

发热及相关症状	
发热	Fever
低热	Hypothermia /Low-grade fever
中度发热	Moderate fever
高热	Hyperthermia / High fever
超高热	Ultra-hyperpyrexia / Extraordinarily high fever
恶性高热	Malignant hyperthermia
感染性发热	Infectious / Septic fever
非感染性	Non-infectious / Aseptic
不明原因发热	Fever of unknown origin, FUO
峰形热	Spiking fever
药物热	Drug fever
稽留热	Continued / Prolonged fever
驰张热	Remittent fever

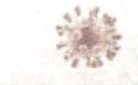

间歇热	Intermittent fever
回归热	Recurring / Relapsing fever
周期热	Periodic fever
不规则热	Irregular fever
升热期	Fervescence period
退热期	Defervescence period
寒战	Shiver
畏寒	Chill
出汗	Sweat / Perspiration
盗汗	Night sweat
冷汗	Cold sweat
淋巴结肿大	Lymphadenopathy/LN enlargement
脓毒血症	Sepsis
导管性脓毒症	Catheter-related sepsis
疼痛症状	
疼痛部位	Location of pain
背痛	Back pain / Backache
腰痛	Flank pain
头痛	Headache
偏头痛	Migraine
丛集性头痛	Cluster headache
胸痛	Chest pain
心前区痛	Substernal pain
心绞痛	Angina
腹痛	Abdominal pain
胃痛	Stomachache

肢体痛	Acrodynia / Pain in limbs
关节痛	Arthralgia / Joint pain
疼痛描述	Pain description
锐痛	Sharp pain
钝痛	Dull pain
刺痛	Twinge / Stabbing pain
酸痛	Ache
绞痛	Colic pain
烧灼痛	Burning pain
反跳痛	Rebound tenderness
压痛	Tenderness
搏动性痛	Throbbing pain
放射性痛	Radiating pain
痉挛性痛	Cramping pain
持续性痛	Constant pain
间歇性痛	Intermittent pain
呼吸系统相关症状	
喷嚏	Sneeze
胸痛	Chest pain
胸闷	Chest tightness
发绀	Cyanosis
指端紫绀	Acrocyanosis
咯血	Hemoptysis
呼吸困难	Dyspnea
心源性呼吸困难	Cardiac dyspnea
吸气性呼吸困难	Inspiratory dyspnea

呼气性呼吸困难	Expiratory dyspnea
混合型呼吸困难	Mixed dyspnea
静息时呼吸困难	Dyspnea at rest
活动时呼吸困难	Dyspnea on exertion
夜间阵发性呼吸困难	Paroxysmal nocturnal dyspnea，PND
端坐呼吸	Orthopnea
三凹征	Chest retractions
呼吸异常	Abnormal respiratory rhythm
频率/深度/节律/幅度	Frequency/Depth/Rhythm/Range
呼吸深度	Respiratory depth
呼吸深快	Hyperpnea
呼吸急促	Tachypnea
呼吸缓慢	Bradypnea
呼吸暂停	Apnea
Kussmaul 呼吸	Kussmaul breathing
浅快呼吸	Rapid shallow breathing
周期性呼吸	Periodic breathing
不规则呼吸	Irregular breathing
潮式呼吸	Tidal breathing
间停呼吸	Biots breathing
叹息样呼吸	Sighing breath
胸腹矛盾呼吸	Paradoxical breathing
咳嗽	Cough
慢性咳嗽	Chronic cough

刺激性咳嗽	Irritable cough
持续性咳嗽	Persistent cough
发作性 / 阵发性咳嗽	Paroxysmal cough
喘咳	Wheezing / Dyspnea with cough
干咳	Dry cough
咳痰	Expectoration / Wet cough
痰量	Sputum quantity
少痰	Scanty sputum
颜色	Color
黄绿色痰	Green-yellowish sputum
铁锈色痰	Rusty sputum
血痰	Bloody sputum
黏稠度	Viscosity
泡沫样痰	Frothy sputum
稀痰	Thin sputum
浓痰	Thick sputum
气味	Smell
脓痰	Purulent sputum
恶臭痰	Fetid sputum
胸部视诊	Inspection
桶状胸	Barrel chest
杵状指	Clubbed finger
胸部触诊	Chest Palpation
胸廓扩张度	Thoracic expansion
触觉震颤	Tactile fremitus

胸膜摩擦感	Pleural friction fremitus
胸廓挤压征	Thoracic compression test
胸部叩诊	Chest percussion
深吸气	Deep breath
屏气	Hold breath
浊音	Dullness
鼓音	Tympanitic note
清音	Resonant note
胸部听诊	Chest auscultation
支气管呼吸音	Bronchial breath sound
肺泡呼吸音	Vesicular breath sound
支气管肺泡呼吸音	Bronchovesicular breath sound
啰音	Rale
干啰音	Dry rale
高调干啰音	Sibilant rhonchi
低调干啰音	Sonorous rhonchi
湿啰音	Crackle / Moist rale
粗湿啰音	Coarse moist rale
中湿啰音	Medium moist rale
细湿啰音	Fine crackle
捻发音	Crepitus
喘鸣	Stridor / Wheeze
喘息	Gasp(ing)
哮鸣音	Wheezing rale
胸膜摩擦音	Pleural friction rub

循环系统及相关症状

动脉	Artery
静脉	Vein
舒张压	Diastolic blood pressure, DBP
收缩压	Systolic blood pressure, SBP
射血分数	Ejection fraction, EF
高血压	Hypertension
低血压	Hypotension
心率	Heart rate
心律	Cardiac rhythm
心音	Heart sound
脉搏	Pulse
心悸	Palpitation
心绞痛	Angina
液体潴留	Fluid retention
心肌顺应性	Myocardial compliance
心脏视诊	Inspection of the heart
心尖搏动移位	Apical impulse displacement
负性心尖搏动	Inward impulse
心脏触诊	Palpation of the heart
心包摩擦感	Pericardium friction rub
震颤	Thrill
心脏叩诊	Percussion of the heart
心浊音界	Cardiac dullness border
心脏听诊	Auscultation of the heart
心脏瓣膜	Heart valve

二尖瓣区	Mitral valve area
肺动脉瓣区	Pulmonary valve area
主动脉瓣区	Aortic valve area
主动脉瓣第二听诊区	The second aortic valve area
三尖瓣区	Tricuspid valve area
心脏杂音	Cardiac murmur
收缩期杂音	Systolic murmur
舒张期杂音	Diastolic murmur
额外心音	Extra cardiac sound
奔马律	Gallop rhythm
开瓣音	Opening snap
心包叩击音	Pericardial knock
收缩期喀喇音	Systolic ejection click / sound
心律失常	Arrhythmia
心动过速	Tachycardia
心动过缓	Bradycardia
心房颤动	Atrial fibrillation
心音分裂	Splitting of heart sounds
血管检查	Examination of blood vessels
水冲脉	Water-hammer pulse
交替脉	Pulsus alternans
奇脉	Paradoxical pulse
脉搏短绌	Pulse deficit
周围血管征	Signs of peripheral vascular disease
枪击音	Pistol shot sound
颈动脉搏动增强	Visible pulsation of carotid artery

血液系统及相关症状

贫血	Anemia
溶血性贫血	Hemolytic anemia
缺铁性贫血	Iron-deficiency anemia
面色苍白	Pale
皮肤干燥	Dry skin
出血	Hemorrhage
瘀点	Petechia
瘀斑	Ecchymosis / Bruise
紫癜	Purpura
渗血	Ooze/Oozing of the blood
血疱	Blood blister
血肿	Hematoma
皮下血肿	Subcutaneous hematoma
鼻出血 / 鼻衄	Epistaxis / Nasal bleed(ing)

泌尿系统及相关症状

急性肾损伤	Acute kidney injury, AKI
尿液	Urine
血尿	Hematuria
无痛性血尿	Painless hematuria
终末血尿	Terminal hematuria
肉眼血尿	Gross hematuria
镜下血尿	Microscopic hematuria
全程血尿	Hematuria in the whole process of urination

一过性血尿	Transient hematuria
排尿	Urinate
夜尿	Nocturia
无尿	Anuria
少尿	Oliguria
多尿	Polyuria
尿频	Frequent urination
尿急	Urgent urination
尿痛	Pain during urination/Urodynia
排尿困难	Dysuria
尿失禁	Urinary incontinence
急迫性尿失禁	Urge urinary incontinence, UUI
压力性尿失禁	Stress urinary incontinence, SUI
溢出性尿失禁	Overflow urinary incontinence
反常性尿失禁	Paradoxical urinary incontinence

消化系统及相关症状

胃肠道	Gastrointestinal
十二指肠	Duodenum
憩室	Diverticulum
肠蠕动	Peristalsis
肠鸣	Bowel sound
肠梗阻	Bowel obstruction
肛门停止排气排便	Cannot pass gas or stool at all
上腹部不适	Epigastric / Upper abdominal discomfort
吞咽困难	Dysphagia / Difficulty in swallowing

厌食	Anorexia
腹胀	Abdominal distention / Abdominal bloating
吸收不良	Malabsorption
胃内容物	Stomach content
胃灼热	Heartburn
胃痛	Stomachache / Pain in stomach
肠绞痛	Colica
脐周痛	Periumbilical pain
嗳酸	Acid reflux
嗳气	Belch / Burp
嗝逆	Hiccup
呕吐	Vomit / Throw up
干呕	Retching / Vomiturition
恶心	Nausea
呃逆	Hiccup
反流	Reflux
消化道出血	Gastrointestinal bleeding
呕血	Hematemesis
便血	Hematochezia
血便	Bloody stool
黑便	Melena / Black stool
柏油样便	Tarry stool
隐血	Occult blood, OB
应激性溃疡	Stress ulcer
胆道出血	Hemobilia

腹腔积血	Hemoperitoneum
排便情况	Bowel movement
排便	Defecate
大便形态	Shape
成形便	Formed stool
硬便	Hard stool
泡沫样便	Frothy stool
稀便	Loose stool
腹泻	Diarrhea
水样泻	Watery diarrhea
黏液泻	Mucous diarrhea
脂肪泻	Fatty diarrhea / Steatorrhea
慢性腹泻	Chronic diarrhea
急性腹泻	Acute diarrhea
难治性腹泻	Intractable diarrhea
便秘	Constipation
功能性便秘	Functional constipation
器质性便秘	Organic constipation
大便失禁	Fecal incontinence
肛门排气	Pass / Release gas by anus
里急后重	Tenesmus
右上腹痛	Right upper quadrant abdominal pain
黄疸	Jaundice
巩膜黄染	Scleral icterus
腹水	Ascites

腹膜刺激征	Signs of peritoneal irritation
压痛	Tenderness
反跳痛	Rebound tenderness
板状腹	Abdominal rigidity

神经精神系统及相关症状

意识障碍	Disturbance of consciousness
嗜睡	Somnolence
意识模糊	Confusion
昏睡	Stupor / Lethargy
昏迷	Coma
谵妄	Delirium
晕厥	Syncope / Faint
倦睡	Drowsiness
神经症状	Neurological symptoms
虚弱（无力）	Muscle weakness
疲乏	Fatigue / lassitude
不适	Discomfort / Malaise
眩晕	Vertigo
抽搐	Tic
手足抽搐	Tetany
惊厥	Convulsion
搔痒	Pruritus / Itch
麻木	Numbness
偏身麻木	Hemianesthesia
蚁走感	Formication

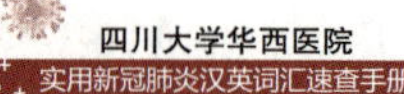

麻刺感	Tingling
痛觉过敏	Hyperpathia / Hyperalgesia
痛觉减退	Hypoalgesia
偏身轻瘫	Hemiplegia
手抖	Hand tremor / shake
脑出血	Intracerebral hemorrhage, ICH
蛛网膜下腔出血	Subarachnoid hemorrhage, SAH
认知障碍	Cognitive dysfunction
记忆力下降	Amnesia / Memory deterioration
计算不能	Dyscalculia
情感障碍	Mood disorder
情感淡漠	Apathy
情感高涨	Elation
欣快	Euphoria
情感不稳	Emotional lability / Mood instability
惊恐	Phobia
焦虑（忧虑）	Anxiety / Agitation
抑郁	Depression
躁狂 / 轻度躁狂	Mania / Hypomania
易激惹性	Irritability / Edginess
精神症状	Mental status
失眠	Insomnia
多梦	Dreaminess
幻觉	Hallucination
妄想	Delusion
错觉	Illusion

内分泌系统及相关症状

消瘦	Emaciation / Underweight
肥胖	Obesity / Overweight
多饮（烦渴）	Polydipsia / Enhanced thirst
多食	Polyphagia
多汗	Excessive sweating / Hyperhidrosis
怕冷	Cold intolerance
怕热	Heat intolerance
水肿	Edema
黏液性水肿	Mucous edema
皮肤色素沉着	Skin pigmentation
心源性水肿	Cardiogenic edema
肾源性水肿	Nephrogenic edema
肝源性水肿	Hepatogenic edema
凹陷性水肿	Pitting edema
非凹陷性水肿	Nonpitting edema
局限性水肿	Localized edema
全身性水肿	Generalized edema / Anasarca

眼及耳鼻咽喉相关症状

眼部症状	Eye symptoms
巩膜黄染	Scleral icterus
结膜炎	Conjunctivitis
瞳孔	Pupil
视物模糊	Blurred vision
流泪	Tear / Lacrimation / Tear secretion

复视	Diplopia / Double vision
斜视	Strabismus
偏盲	Hemianopia
异物感	Foreign body sensation
失明	Vision loss / lose vision
视力减退	Declined vision /Loss of vision
眼痛	Eye pain
畏光	Photophobia
耳鼻咽喉症状	ENT symptoms
鼻咽的	Nasopharyngeal
嗅觉减退	Hyposmia
嗅觉丧失	Anosmia
鼻塞	Nasal congestion
鼻干燥	Dry nose
鼻涕	Rhinorrhea / Runny nose
打喷嚏	Sneeze
鼻出血 / 鼻衄	Epistaxis / Nasal bleed(ing)
打鼾	Snore
口咽的	Oropharyngeal
流涎	Drool
声嘶	Hoarseness
发音困难	Dysphonia
咽痛	Pharyngeal pain / Pharyngalgia
吞咽痛	Painful swallowing / Odynophagia
咽喉痛	Sore throat
喉头水肿	Laryngeal edema

舌后坠	Glossoptosis
听力减退	Hearing loss
耳聋	Deafness
耳痛	Otalgia / Ear pain
耳鸣	Tinnitus

第四章　既往史及家族史

既往史

无药物过敏史
No known drug allergies， NKDA
不详
Unknown
健康状况佳（差）
General health status was good (poor).
否认既往心、肺疾病史
Deny history of cardiovascular or pulmonary disease
……年前曾患过……
Had... ...years ago
易患……
Be susceptible to... .
手术史
History of surgery
……时候因……行……手术
... was done in ... due to ...
手术并发症
surgical complications
外伤史
history of trauma
预防接种史
immunization records
对……过敏
Be allergic to ... / Have allergy to ...

个人及家庭史

出生于（出生地）	Was born in / Birthplace
出生后一直生活于	Lived in / at ... since birth
文盲	Unable to read or write / Illiterate
受教育程度	Education background
宗教信仰	Religious belief
职业	Occupation
退休	Retirement
经济情况	Financial status
兵役	Military service
卫生习惯	Hygiene habit
不洁性交史	High-risk sexual behavior
物质依赖	Substance dependence
吸食大麻	Take marijuana/Weed
不吸烟	No smoking
以……频率抽烟……	Have smoked ... (daily / every other day / once a week ...)
戒烟	Stop / Quit smoking
不饮酒	No alcohol
偶而饮酒	Drink occasionally
过度饮酒	Drink heavily
每天饮（酒 1 升）……	Drink xx(1L of wine / liquor) daily
饮食偏好	Food preference
饮食禁忌	Dietary restriction
运动频率	Frequency of exercise
生活压力	Life pressure

遗传疾病	Genetic / hereditary / inherited disease
没有……家族史	Has no family history of ...
死因	Cause of death
健在	Be alive and well

月经婚育史

未婚	Single
已婚	Married
结婚年龄	Age of marriage
配偶的健康状况	Health status of spouse
初潮年龄	Age of menarche
月经周期	Menstrual cycle
行经期	Menstrual period
末次月经时间	Last menstrual period, LMP
绝经年龄	Age of menopause
白带异常	Abnormal leucorrhea
经前疼痛	Premenstrual pain
痛经	Pain during the menstruation / Dysmenorrhea
怀孕和生产次数	Pregnancies and labors
流产	Miscarriage / Abortion
剖腹产	Caesarean / C-Section
早产（儿）	Preterm birth, PTB
自然分娩	Natural delivery / Spontaneous labor
产钳分娩	Forceps delivery
产后子痫	Postpartum eclampsia

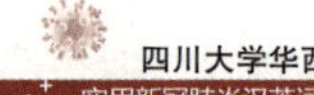

先兆子痫	Preeclampsia
发育正常	Normal development
发育异常（停顿、缺陷、畸形）	Developmental anomaly (arrest, defect, deformity)
发育迟缓	Growth retardation
母乳喂养	Breast feeding
人工喂养	Formula feeding

第五章　常用检查检验

新冠肺炎病原学检查

核酸检测	Nucleic acid test
唾液	Saliva
鼻咽拭子	Nasopharyngeal swab
口咽拭子	Oropharyngeal swab
眼结膜拭子	Conjunctive swab
肛拭子	Anal swab
植绒拭子	Flocked swab
采样液（固定液）	Sampling solution
粪便标本	Feces / Stool specimen
试剂盒	Kit
痰检查	Sputum examination
痰液收集杯	Sputum collection cup
吸痰	Sputum suction / Aspiration
负压吸引器	Vacuum suction
气道分泌物	Respiratory tract secretion, RTS
密闭无菌容器	Airtight sterile container
支气管镜检查	Bronchoscopy
纤维支气管镜检查	Fibro bronchoscopy
支气管灌洗液	Bronchial lavage fluid
肺泡灌洗液	Alveolar lavage fluid
气管隆突	Carina of trachea
肺门	Hilar
抽血	Draw blood

血标本	Blood sample
血浆	Plasma
血清标本	Serum specimen
抗凝采血管	Anticoagulant tube
蓝头管	Blue-top tube
粉头管（合血管）	Pink-top tube
查血型	ABO typing
合血	Cross-match
输血科	Dept. of blood transfusion
血库	Blood bank

医技检查

胸部 CT	Chest CT
增强 CT 扫描	Enhanced CT scan
高分辨率 CT	High-resolution computed tomography, HRCT
核磁共振成像	Magnetic resonance imaging, MRI
正电子发射计算机断层扫描	Positron emission tomography, PET
支气管造影	Bronchography
纤维支气管镜检查	Fibro bronchoscopy
肺穿刺（活检）	Pulmonary biopsy
胸腔穿刺	Thoracentesis
心电图	Electrocardiogram, ECG/EKG
超声心动图	Echocardiography, ECG / Echo
腹部彩超	Abdominal ultrasonography

超声内镜	Endoscopic ultrasonography, EUS
胃镜检查	Gastroscopy
肠镜检查	Enteroscopy
经内镜逆行性胰胆管造影术	Endoscopic retrograde cholangiopancreatography, ERCP

实验室检查

宏基因组测序	Metagenomic next-generation sequencing, mNGS
酶联免疫吸附试验	Enzyme linked immunosorbent assay, ELISA
逆转录 PCR	Reverse transcription PCR
待查	Yet to be investigated
基因组测序	Genome sequencing
病毒载量	Viral load
炎性指标	Inflammatory indicators
浓度	Concentration
心肌酶	Myocardial enzymes
血沉	Erythrocyte sedimentation rate, ESR
细胞因子检测	Cytokines test
血常规	Blood routine / Complete blood count, CBC
淋巴细胞	Lymphocyte
绝对淋巴细胞计数	Absolute lymphocyte count, ALC
淋巴细胞减少	Lymphocytopenia
红细胞计数	Erythrocyte count
红细胞压积	Hematocrit

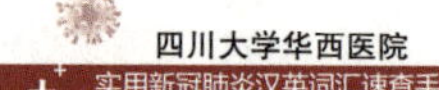
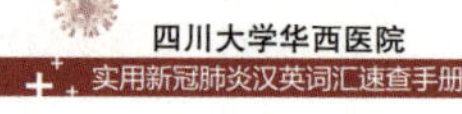

网织红细胞计数	Reticulocyte count
血红蛋白	Hemoglobin
中性分叶（杆状）核粒细胞	Segmented neutrophils
中性粒细胞	Neutrophils
嗜酸性粒细胞	Eosinophils
嗜碱性粒细胞	Basophils
单核细胞	Monocytes
巨噬细胞	Macrophage
白细胞减少	Leukopenia
白细胞增多	Leukocytosis
血小板计数	Platelet count
血生化	Blood biochemistry
总蛋白	Total protein, TP
白蛋白	Albumin
球蛋白	Globulin
血糖	Blood glucose
钠	Sodium
钾	Potassium
氯	Chloride
钙	Calcium
镁	Magnesium
肌酐清除率	Creatinine(Cr) clearance
尿素氮	Blood urea nitrogen, BUN
糖化血红蛋白 A1c	Glycosylated hemoglobin A1c, HbA1c
血栓弹力图	Thromboelastography, TEG

凝血图	Coagulation profile, Coags
血浆凝血酶原时间	Prothrombin time, PT
活化部分凝血活酶时间	Activated partial thromboplastin time, APTT
纤维蛋白原	Fibrinogen, FB
D-二聚体	D-dimer

致病微生物

新冠肺炎病毒	SARS-CoV-2
冠状病毒	Coronavirus
副流感病毒	Parainfluenza virus
流感病毒	Influenza virus
腺病毒	Adenovirus
鼻病毒	Rhinovirus
人偏肺病毒	Human metapneumovirus, HMPV
呼吸道合胞病毒	Respiratory syncytial virus, RSV
衣原体	Chlamydia
支原体	Mycoplasma
b 型流感嗜血杆菌	Hemophilus influenzae type b, Hib
革兰氏阳性球菌	Gram-positive cocci
革兰氏阴性杆菌	Gram-negative bacilli
鲍曼不动杆菌	*Acinetobacter baumannii*, AB
铜绿假单胞菌	*Pseudomonas aeruginosa*, PA
耐甲氧西林金黄色葡萄球菌	Methicillin-resistant *Staphylococcus aureus*, MRSA
耐万古霉素金黄色葡萄球菌	Vancomycin-resistant *Staphylococcus aureus*, VRSA

耐万古霉素肠球菌	Vancomycin-resistant enterococci, VRE
超广谱 β－内酰胺酶	Extended-spectrum β-lactamase, ESBLs
耐碳青霉烯类肺炎克雷伯杆菌	Carbapenem-resistant klebsiella pneumoniae, CRKP
产气荚膜梭菌	Clostridium perfringen

血气分析

氧分压	Partial pressure of oxygen, PaO_2
二氧化碳分压	Partial pressure of carbon dioxide, $PaCO_2$
二氧化碳总量	Total carbon dioxide, TCO_2
肺泡每分通气量	Alveolar minute ventilation
呼气末正压	Positive end-expiratory pressure, PEEP
潮气量	Tidal volume
血氧饱和度	Oxygen saturation, SaO_2
氧合指数	Oxygenation index
酸碱	acid-base
标准碳酸氢盐	Standard bicarbonate, SB
实际碳酸氢盐	Actual bicarbonate, AB
剩余碱	Base excess, BE

大小便检查

尿常规	Urinalysis
渗透压	Osmotic pressure / Osmolality
尿比重	Urine specific gravity
管型	Cast
蛋白肌酐比	Protein to creatinine ratio

粪便标本	Feces / Stool specimen
性状	Property
黏液	Mucus
隐血	Occult blood, OB
寄生虫虫卵	Parasite egg

第六章　胸部影像学检查及诊断

胸部结构

骨性胸廓	Bony thorax
肋骨	Rib
锁骨	Clavicle
胸骨	Sternum
胸骨柄	Sternal manubrium
气管	Trachea
支气管	Bronchus
肺	Lung
肺野	Lung field
肺门	Hilar
肺叶	Pulmonary lobe
肺小叶	Lung lobule
小叶间隔	Interlobular septum
斜裂	Oblique fissure
水平裂	Horizontal fissure
胸膜	Pleura
胸膜下	Subpleural
纵隔	Mediastinum
肺门淋巴结	Hilar lymph node
横膈	Diaphragm
胸腺	Thymus
食管	Esophagus

胸部 X 光

前后位投影	Anteroposterior projection, AP
后前位投影	Posteroanterior projection, PA
侧位投影	Lateral projection
立位投影	Upright projection
斜位投影	Oblique projection
右前斜位投影	Right anterior oblique projection, RAO
左前斜位投影	Left anterior oblique projection, LAO
前后斜位投影	Anteroposterior oblique projection
前凸位投影	Lordotic position projection
轴位投影	Axial projection
头位投影	Cranial projection
尾位投影	Caudal projection
胸部透视	Chest fluoroscopy

胸部 CT 诊断用语

层厚	Slice thickness
肺窗	Lung window
纵隔窗	Mediastinal window
肺部征象	Pulmonary pattern
单侧 / 双侧 / 弥漫性	Unilateral / Bilateral / Diffuse
外周分布	Peripheral distribution
中央分布	Central distribution
沿支气管血管束	Peribronchovascular distribution
间质性	Interstitial
密度	Density

磨玻璃影	Ground-glass opacification, GGO
圆形 / 结节样影	Rounded / Nodular shadow
斑片影	Patchy infiltrates
铺路石征	Crazy paving appearance
白肺	White lung
间质纤维化	Interstitial fibrosis
细网格状影	Fine reticular opacities
小叶间隔增厚	Interlobular septal thickening
反向晕轮征 / 环礁征	Reverse halo sign / Atoll sign
空气支气管造影片	Air bronchogram
支气管扩张	Bronchiectasis
血管壁增厚	Vascular wall thickening
肺部病变	Pulmonary lesions
气管狭窄与闭塞	Tracheal stenosis and obstruction
肺实变	Pulmonary consolidation
肺气肿	Emphysema
肺不张	Atelectasis
钙化	Calcification
结节	Nodule
肿块	Mass
空腔与空洞	Air containing space and cavity
肺间质病变	Interstitial Lung disease, ILD
纤维化	Fibrosis
肺间质纤维化	Pulmonary interstitial fibrosis
胸腔积液	Pleural effusion
气胸	Pneumothorax

液气胸	Hydropneumothorax
胸膜增厚	Pleural thickening
淋巴结肿大	Lymphadenopathy
纵隔淋巴结肿大	Mediastinal lymphadenopathy
人工智能	Artificial intelligence

CT 诊断描述

双肺间质纤维化
Interstitial fibrosis in both lungs
多发肺大泡
Multiple pulmonary bullae
纵膈淋巴结肿大
Mediastinal lymphadenopathy
多发磨玻璃小斑片影
Multiple patchy-like ground glass opacities
双肺散在斑片、条片、条索状磨玻璃影
Diffuse patches, strips, and cord-like ground glass opacification in both lungs
双肺多发磨玻璃影
Multiple ground glass shadows in both lungs
双肺下叶实变影
Consolidation in the Inferior lobes of both lungs
支气管轻度扩张
Mild bronchiectasis
右肺中叶见纤维化条索状影
Fibrous streak shadow observed in middle lobe of right lung

少许纤维条索影
A few fibrous cord
小结节、钙化灶、斑片条索影
Small nodules, calcifications, and patchy cord-like shadow
部分支气管壁增厚
Partial thickening of the bronchial wall
肺气肿
Emphysema

CT 肺部定位

右肺中叶
Right middle lobe
左肺上叶下舌段
Left upper lung lobe inferior lingular segment
病变以内、中带分布为主。
The lesions are mainly distributed in the inner and middle zones.
病变以肺野外带为主。
The lesions are mainly distributed in lung peripheral zones.

CT 检查意见

合并感染可能
Possibility of concurrent / combined infection
考虑双肺感染性病变
Infectious lesions of both lungs should be considered.
考虑炎症导致
Probably caused by inflammation

第七章　常见疾病诊断

呼吸系统

肺部感染	Pulmonary infection
急性上呼吸道感染	Acute upper respiratory tract infection, AURTI
普通感冒	Common cold
流行性感冒	Influenza
肺炎	Pneumonia
新型冠状病毒肺炎	COVID-19
病毒性肺炎	Viral pneumonia
细菌性肺炎	Bacterial pneumonia
支原体肺炎	Mycoplasma pneumonia
社区获得性肺炎	Community-acquired pneumonia, CAP
医院获得性肺炎	Hospital-acquired pneumonia, HAP
呼吸机相关性肺炎	Ventilator-associated pneumonia, VAP
不明原因肺炎	Unexplained pneumonia
限制性通气功能障碍	Restrictive ventilatory disorder(dysfunction)
慢性阻塞性肺疾病	Chronic obstructive pulmonary disease, COPD
支气管炎	Bronchitis
支气管扩张	Bronchiectasis
急性呼吸窘迫综合征	Acute respiratory distress syndrome, ARDS
呼吸衰竭	Respiratory failure
低氧血症	Hypoxemia

顽固性低氧血症	Refractory hypoxemia
二氧化碳潴留	Hypercapnia / CO_2 retention
呼吸性酸中毒	Respiratory acidosis
呼吸性碱中毒	Respiratory alkalosis
肺栓塞	Pulmonary embolism
静脉栓塞	Venous embolism
深静脉血栓	Deep vein thrombosis, DVT
栓子	Embolus
哮喘	Asthma
心源性哮喘	Cardiac asthma
支气管性哮喘	Bronchial asthma
肺气肿	Emphysema
肺水肿	Pulmonary edema
心源性肺水肿	Cardiogenic pulmonary edema
肺实变	Pulmonary consolidation
肺不张	Atelectasis
胸水 / 胸腔积液	Pleural effusion / Hydrothorax
漏出液	Transudate
渗出液	Exudate
气胸	Pneumothorax
血胸	Hemothorax
上气道梗阻	Upper airway obstruction, UAO
肺间质纤维化	Pulmonary interstitial fibrosis
空泡征	Vacuole sign
肺癌	Lung cancer
肺结核	Pulmonary tuberculosis

心血管系统

心血管疾病	Cardiovascular disease
冠心病	Coronary artery disease, CAD
动脉粥样硬化	Atherosclerosis
急性冠状动脉综合征	Acute coronary syndrome, ACS
心肌梗塞	Myocardial infarction
ST 段抬高的心肌梗塞	ST-elevation myocardial infarction, STEMI
非 ST 段抬高的心肌梗塞	Non-ST elevation myocardial infarction, NSTEMI
高血压	Hypertension
心肌重构	Cardiac remodeling
心室增大	Ventricular hypertrophy
心房增大	Atrium hypertrophy
心脏瓣膜病	Valvular heart disease, VHD
二尖瓣狭窄	Mitral stenosis, MS
二尖瓣返流	Mitral regurgitation
二尖瓣关闭不全	Mitral regurgitation, MR
三尖瓣关闭不全	Tricuspid regurgitation, TR
主动脉瓣狭窄	Aortic stenosis, AS
主动脉瓣关闭不全	Aortic regurgitation, AR
心力衰竭	Heart failure
急性心力衰竭	Acute heart failure
慢性心力衰竭	Chronic heart failure

肺动脉高压	Pulmonary arterial hypertension, PAH
右心功能不全	Right ventricle dysfunction
心律失常	Cardiac arrhythmia
心动过速	Tachycardia
心动过缓	Bradycardia
期前收缩	Premature beats
窦性	Sinus
房室的	Atrioventricular
阵发性	Paroxysmal
心房颤动	Atrial fibrillation
心房扑动	Atrial flutter
室性心动过速	Ventricular tachycardia
尖端扭转性室速	Torsades de pointes, TDP
心室颤动	Ventricular fibrillation
房室传导阻滞	Atrioventricular block
心包填塞	Cardiac tamponade
心包积液	Pericardial effusion / Hydropericardium
心包积血	Hemopericardium
风湿性心脏病	Rheumatic heart disease
感染性心内膜炎	Infective endocarditis, IE
病毒性心肌炎	Viral myocarditis
先天性心脏病	Congenital heart disease, CHD
肥厚型心肌病	Hypertrophic cardiopathy, HCM

感染性疾病

继发细菌感染	Secondary bacterial infection

导管相关性血流感染	Catheter-associated bloodstream infection
多重耐药菌	Multiple drug resistant (MDR) bacteria
器官功能障碍	Organ dysfunction
流感	Influenza
结核	Tuberculosis
休克	Shock
分布性休克	Distributive shock
感染性休克	Septic shock
心源性休克	Cardiogenic shock
梗阻性休克	Obstructive shock

血液系统

凝血功能障碍	Coagulopathy
缺铁性贫血	Iron-deficiency anemia
溶血性贫血	Hemolytic anemia
地中海贫血	Thalassemia
再生障碍性贫血	Aplastic anemia
白血病	Leukemia
脾功能亢进	Hypersplenism
紫癜	Purpura
弥漫性血管内凝血	Disseminated intravascular coagulation, DIC

泌尿系统

急性肾损伤	Acute kidney injury, AKI
慢性肾病	Chronic Kidney Disease, CKD

急性肾小球肾炎	Acute glomerulonephritis
肾病综合征	Nephrotic syndrome
尿路感染	Urinary tract infection, UTI
高钠血症	Hypernatremia
低钾血症	Hypokalemia

消化系统

消化性溃疡	Peptic ulcer
胃溃疡	Gastric ulcer, GU
十二指肠溃疡	Duodenal ulcer, DU
消化道出血	Gastrointestinal bleeding
胃炎	Gastritis
急性化脓性阑尾炎	Acute suppurative appendicitis
腹膜炎	Peritonitis
肝炎	Hepatitis
脂肪性肝病	Fatty liver disease
酒精性肝炎	Alcoholic hepatitis
肝硬化	Hepatic cirrhosis
肝功能损害	Liver dysfunction
胆囊结石	Gallstone
慢性胆囊炎	Chronic cholecystitis
胆总管结石	Choledocholithiasis
急性梗阻化脓性胆管炎	Acute obstructive suppurative cholangitis, AOSC
胰腺炎	Pancreatitis

内分泌系统

甲状腺功能亢进症	Hyperthyroidism
甲状腺功能减退症	Hypothyroidism
甲状腺炎	Thyroiditis
甲状腺癌	Thyroid cancer
库欣综合征	Cushing syndrome
尿崩症	Diabetes insipidus, DI
垂体瘤	Pituitary tumor
嗜铬细胞瘤	Pheochromocytoma
糖尿病	Diabetes mellitus, DM
低血糖症	Hypoglycemia
肥胖	Obesity/Overweight
血脂异常	Dyslipidemia
高尿酸血症	Hyperuricemia, HUA

神经系统

脑疝	Brain herniation
脑水肿	Brain edema
脑出血	Intracerebral hemorrhage, ICH
颅内压增高	Intracranial hypertension
脑膜炎	Meningitis
阿尔茨海默病	Alzheimer’s disease, AD
帕金森病	Parkinson disease, PD
癫痫	Epilepsy
偏头痛	Migraine
紧张性头痛	Tension headache

三叉神经痛	Trigeminal neuralgia, TN
神经胶质瘤	Glioma
脑膜瘤	Meningioma

精神疾病

重性抑郁障碍	Major depressive disorder, MDD
焦虑	Anxiety
强迫障碍	Obsessive-compulsive disorder, OCD
精神分裂症	Schizophrenia
创伤后应激障碍	Post-traumatic stress disorder, PTSD

眼科

结膜炎	Conjunctivitis
角膜炎	Keratitis
巩膜炎	Scleritis
白内障	Cataract
青光眼	Glaucoma
复视	Diplopia/Double vision
高眼压症	Ocular hypertension

耳鼻咽喉

外耳道炎	Otitis externa
中耳炎	Otitis media
耳鸣	Tinnitus
鼻窦炎	Rhinosinusitis
鼻炎	Rhinitis

慢性咽炎	Chronic pharyngitis
嗅觉障碍	Olfactory dysfunction
嗅觉丧失	Anosmia

骨骼肌肉系统

骨折	Fracture
脱位	Dislocation
先天性畸形	Congenital malformation
骨关节炎	Osteoarthritis, OA
类风湿性关节炎	Rheumatoid arthritis, RA
股骨头坏死	Necrosis of the femoral head
颈椎病	Cervical spondylosis
腰椎间盘突出症	Lumbar disc herniation
骨与关节结核	Bone and joint tuberculosis
骨质疏松症	Osteoporosis, OP

第八章　治疗及护理

疾病阶段

病历号	Medical record number
知情同意书	Informed consent
整体情况	General status
潜伏期	Incubation period
无症状感染	Asymptomatic infection
恢复期	Recovery phase
急性期	Acute phase
病危	Critical / Imminence
不稳定	Unstable
稳定	Stable
一般	Fair
液体过负荷	Fluid overload
灌注不足	Inadequate perfusion
脱水	Dehydrated
压力性损伤	Pressure ulcer
深静脉血栓	Deep vein thrombosis, DVT
抗生素过敏	Allergy to antibiotics
简要情况	Briefing
出院	Discharge
急诊	Emergent / Urgent care clinic
对症治疗	Symptomatic treatment
支持性治疗	Supportive care
抢救治疗	Salvage treatment

姑息治疗	Palliative treatment

护理相关

医嘱	Physician's orders
不需要	N/A (non-apply)
护理常规	Routine nursing procedures
一级护理	Grade I nursing
晨间（夜间）护理	Morning (evening) care
监护	Monitoring
生命体征	Vital signs
脉搏血氧仪	Pulse oximeter
心电监护	Cardiac monitoring
呼吸频率	Respiratory rate
平均动脉压	Mean arterial pressure, MAP
血压监测	Blood pressure monitoring
血糖监测	Blood glucose monitoring
尿量	Urine output
每 6 小时一次	Every 6 hours (q6h)
活动状态	Activity
卧床休息	Bed rest / Rest-cure
俯卧位	Prone position / Lie on the stomach
抬高床头（尾）	Raise the head (foot) of the bed
随意活动	Move freely
病房内活动	Move in the ward
每 2 小时更换体位	Change position q2h
体位引流	Postural drainage

护理项目	Nursing item
留置导尿	Reserved urethral catheter / Indwelling catheterization
记 24h 出入量	Daily I/O (intake and output)
预防褥疮	Prevent from bedsore
深静脉血栓高危	High risk for DVT
弹力袜	Compression stockings
间歇式气压治疗	Intermittent pneumatic compression, IPC
褥疮护理	Bedsore care
口腔护理	Oral care
胸部物理治疗	Chest physical treatment, CPT or Chest PT
硫酸镁	Magnesium sulphate, $MgSO_4$
用硫酸镁湿敷	Wet compress by $MgSO_4$
目标温度管理	Target temperature management
酒精擦浴	Alcohol sponge bath
保温	Keep warm
冰帽降温	Lower temperature by icecap
冷（热）敷	Apply an ice or a warm pack

饮食及营养

水电解质平衡	Fluid and electrolyte balance
肠道微生态平衡	Gut microbiota balance
营养支持	Nutrition support
饮食方式	Diets
普食	Full diet

禁食	Fasting (NOP, nothing by mouth)
清流质饮食	Clear liquid diet
流质（半流质）饮食	Liquid (Semi-liquid) diet
软食	Soft diet / Soft foods
低盐低脂饮食	Low-salt and low-fat diet
低钠饮食	Low-sodium diet
低嘌呤饮食	Low-purine diet
少（无）渣饮食	Low (Non)-residue diet
高热量饮食	High-caloric diet
高蛋白饮食	High-protein (protein-rich) diet
糖尿病饮食	Diabetic diet
碳水化合物	Carbohydrate
营养供给方式	Feeding patterns
鼻饲	Nasal feeding
肠内营养	Enteral nutrition
肠外营养	Parenteral nutrition
全肠外营养	Total parenteral nutrition, TPN

气道管理

给氧方式	Oxygen administration
鼻导管	Nasal cannula / tube
人工球囊呼吸器	Ambu bag
面罩氧疗	Mask oxygen therapy
普通面罩	Standard mask
文丘里面罩	Venturi mask

储氧面罩	Non-rebreather mask, NRB
球囊面罩	Bag-Valve-Mask, BVM
氧流量	Oxygen flux
吸氧（2~4 升 / 分）	O_2 inhalation (2-4 L/min)
吸氧浓度	Fraction of inspired oxygen, FiO_2
高流量氧疗	High flow oxygen therapy
高流量鼻导管	High-flow nasal cannula, HFNC
雾化吸入	Aerosol inhalation
雾化器	Nebulizer
雾化	Nebulization
湿化	Humidification
湿化瓶	Humidification bottle
祛痰	Remove / Clear sputum
稀化痰液	Loosen mucus

呼吸支持

气道阻力	Airway resistance
保持气道通畅	Keep the airway open
呼吸支持操作	Respiration support
吸痰	Sputum suction
气管吸痰	Tracheal aspiration
镇痛	Analgesia / Reduce pain
镇静	Sedation
肌松药	Muscle relaxant
气管插管	Tracheal intubation
气管切开	Tracheotomy

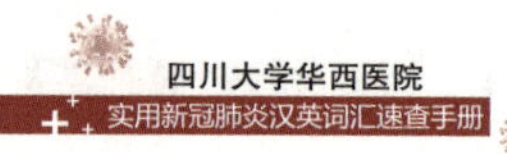

人工肺 / 体外膜肺氧合	Extracorporeal membrane oxygenation, ECMO
胸腔闭式引流	Closed chest drainage / chest tube
深吸气末屏气	Deep inspiration breath hold
水封	Water seal
撤机	Weaning
呼吸肌锻炼	Respiratory muscle training, RMT
肺复张	Lung recruitment
拔管	Extubation
通气方式	Ventilation
插管前的人工通气	Manual ventilation before intubation
俯卧位通气	Prone-position ventilation
机械通气	Mechanical ventilation
无创通气	Non-invasive ventilation
有创通气	Invasive ventilation
喉罩	Laryngeal mask
人工鼻	Artificial nose
一次性呼吸回路	Disposable ventilator circuit
密闭性检测	Airtightness test
呼吸机参数	Ventilator control parameter
持续气道正压	Continuous positive airway pressure, CPAP
气道峰压	Peak inspiratory pressure, PIP
平台压	Plateau pressure, Pplat
潮气量	Tidal volume, TV
肺顺应性	Pulmonary compliance

跨肺压	Transpulmonary pressure
辅助 / 控制模式	Assist-Control (A/C) mode
容量控制通气	Volume-controlled ventilation, VCV
压力支持通气	Pressure support ventilation, PSV
同步间歇指令通气	Synchronized intermittent mandatory ventilation, SIMV
呼气末正压	Positive end-expiratory pressure, PEEP
转运呼吸机	Transport ventilator

循环支持

液体复苏	Fluid resuscitation
心肺复苏	Cardiopulmonary resuscitation, CPR
中心静脉置管	Central venous catheter, CVC
动脉有创血压	Invasive intra-arterial blood pressure
脉搏指数连续心输出量监测	Pulse-induced Contour Cardiac Output, PiCCO
输血	Blood transfusion
晶体液	Crystalloid solution
胶体液	Colloidal solution
血管阻力	Vascular resistance
微循环	Microcirculation
血流动力学	Hemodynamics
液体平衡状态	Fluid balance
容量	Capacity

血液净化

恢复期血浆治疗	Convalescent plasma therapy
血液透析	Hemodialysis
腹膜透析	Peritoneal dialysis
血浆置换	Therapeutic plasma exchange, TPE/ Plasmapheresis
体外血液净化技术	Extracorporeal blood purification technique
连续性肾脏替代治疗	Continuous renal replacement therapy, CRRT

抗感染治疗

怀疑感染的部位	Suspected infection site
皮试（阴性）	Negative skin test reaction
过敏史阴性	No known allergies, NKA
不良反应	Adverse effect, AE
细菌培养	Bacterial culture
需氧菌	Aerobe
厌氧菌	Anaerobe
病原体	Pathogen
治疗方式	Therapy pattern
抗生素医嘱	Antibiotic order
药名 + 剂量 + 途径 + 次数	Drug+ dose+ route +frequency
抗菌药物治疗	Antibacterial drug treatment
抗病毒治疗	Antiviral treatment
预防性用药	Preventive medication
经验性治疗	Empiric therapy

常见交流用语

问候
Greeting
您好！
Hi, how are you?
自我介绍
Self-introduction
我是 XX，是您的主管护士。
I am XX, your nurse on this shift.
身份核查
Patient confirmation
请问您的姓名是？
Your name, please?
请问您的住院号是？
Your ID, please?
询问病情
Inquire about condition
您现在感觉怎么样？
How are you feeling now?
你昨晚睡得好吗？
Did you sleep well last night?
心理安慰
Psychological care
放轻松。
Relax.

不要紧张。
Don't be nervous.
如果有不适，请及时告知我们。
If you don’t feel comfy/comfortable, please let us know.
您的精神看起来好多了。
You look much better.
祝您早日康复！
Hope you will recover soon.

常见护理操作分解

测生命体征
Check vital signs
测脉搏
Check the pulse
我将为您测脉搏，请将手给我。
I am going to check your pulse. Please give me your hand.
测体温
Check the temperature
我将为您测体温，请将体温计夹在腋下至少 5 分钟。
I am going to take your temperature. Please hold the thermometer under your armpit for at least 5 minutes.
测血压
Check blood pressure
我将为您测血压，请平躺，保持手臂不动。
I am going to take your blood pressure. Please lie down and keep the arm still.

氧饱和度监测
Oxygen saturation monitoring
我将为您进行氧饱和度监测。
I am going to check your O_2 sat [O-two sat].
请把手给我 / 请伸出手。
Please reach out your hand.
测血糖
Check blood sugar.
我将为您测血糖。
I am going to check your blood sugar.
请将手掌摊开，保持不动。
Palm up and hold for a while, please.
请用棉签按压针眼处至少 1 分钟，彻底止血。
Please hold the swab at least 1 minute until bleeding stops.
抽血
Draw blood
我将为您抽血。
I am going to draw some blood.
请保持手臂不动。
Please keep your arm still.
请捏紧拳头。
Please make a fist.
请松开拳头。
Please release your hand.
请按压止血。
Please press the puncture site until bleeding stops.

取咽拭子
Throat swab collection
我将为您取咽拭子标本。
I am going to collect a throat swab.
请用清水漱口。
Please rinse your mouth with water.
（经口）请张嘴发“啊”音，并保持不动。
Open your mouth and keep saying “ah”.
（经鼻）请仰头，并保持不动。
Please keep your head up.
在开始前请擤鼻涕。
Please blow your nose before I start.
大便标本采集
Stool sample collection
您需要留取大便标本做实验室检查。
We need you to collect a stool sample for lab tests.
这是您的大便标本盒。
This is your stool sample container.
采集大便标本时请不要与尿液混合及触碰到其他地方。
Try not to collect urine or contact somewhere else when collecting a stool sample.
标本装满盒子的 1/3 即可。
Fill around a third of the container.
尿标本采集
Urine specimen collection

您需要留取尿标本做实验室检查。

We need you to collect a urine sample for lab tests.

请拿好您的尿标本采集杯。

This is your urine sample container.

请直接将尿液解在标本杯中，留取中段尿效果最佳。

Urinate directly into the container. Try to keep the mid-stream urine.

请尽量留取清晨第一次尿液。

Keep the first urine in the morning.

尿标本留取后请在 1 小时内送检。

Please hand in your urine sample for test within 1 hour.

拍背

Chest percussion

我将为您拍背，协助您咳出痰液。

I am going to lightly tap your back to help you cough up the sputum.

请取俯卧位。

Please lie on your stomach.

吸痰

Sputum suction

我将为您进行吸痰操作。

I am doing mucus suction for you.

（经口吸痰）请保持张嘴，并放松。

Keep your mouth open and relax.

（经鼻吸痰）请将头稍微后仰，并放松。

Tilt your head slightly back and relax.

氧疗
Oxygen therapy
我将为您进行氧疗。
I am going to put you on oxygen therapy.
我将为您带上鼻导管 / 面罩。
Let me put on the nasal tube/facial mask for you.
请用鼻子呼吸，勿用嘴呼吸。
Please breathe through your nose instead of your mouth.
佩戴呼吸机
Wear ventilator
我将为您佩戴呼吸机，请采取半卧位。
I am going to set up the respirator for you. Please be half-seated.
呼吸机参数已调整好，我将为您佩戴鼻罩 / 面罩。
The ventilator is ready. Now let me put on the mask for you.
呼吸机会自动感应来帮助您减轻气紧症状。
The machine will adapt to your breath and make you feel more comfortable.
雾化治疗
Use a nebulizer
我将协助您进行雾化治疗。
I am going to help you with the nebulizer.
请选择您觉得舒适的坐姿。
Please find a comfortable seated position.
请含住口含器。
Keep your lips firm around the mouthpiece.

用嘴吸气直至吸尽药物，用鼻子呼气。
Inhale through your mouth until the medicine is used, and exhale through your nose.
完成雾化后请用清水漱口和清洁面部。
When you finish, rinse your mouth with water and clean your face.
静脉输液
Intravenous infusion
我将为您进行静脉输液。
I am going to administer an iv for you.
请捏紧拳头，我将选择一处合适的静脉血管进行穿刺。
Please make a fist. I am going to select a suitable puncture site.
请松开拳头。
Please release your fist.
请保持手臂不动，我将用敷贴对穿刺点进行固定 。
Please hold while I'm fixing the puncture site with the plaster.
肌肉注射
Intramuscular injection
我将为您进行肌肉注射。
I am going to give you an intramuscular injection.
请取侧卧位。
Please lie on one side.
请用棉签按压针眼处 5 分钟，彻底止血。
Apply some pressure at the puncture site with the swab at least 5 minutes until bleeding stops.
安置尿管
Urinary catheterization

我将为您安置尿管。
I am going to place a forley catheter for you.
请分开双腿，深呼吸，保持不动。
Please open your legs. Take a deep breath and hold still.
我将对会阴部位进行消毒，然后安置尿管。
I'm sterilizing your genital area first, then insert the foley.
可能会有一点刺痛感。请深呼吸，尽量放松。
There may be a little bit pain. Take a deep breath and try to relax.
更换床单
Bedding change
我将为您更换床上用品。
I am going to change your beddings.
血液透析
Hemodialysis
我将为您做血液透析。
I am going to do hemodialysis for you.
保持这只手不要动。
Don't move this arm.
我将为您测量血压和脉搏。
I am going to check your blood pressure and pulse.
您现在感觉怎么样？
How are you feeling now?
如果有不舒服，请马上呼叫我们。
Please let us know if you feel uncomfortable.

口腔护理
Oral care
我将为您进行口腔护理。
I am going to give you some oral care.
请张开嘴，我将使用棉球清洁您的口腔。
Open your mouth. I am going to swab your mouth.
操作中若有不适，请向我们示意。
Please let us know if you don’t feel well during the procedure.
尿管护理
Foley care
我要检查一下您的尿管。
I am going to check your catheter.
请放松，我将进行消毒。
Please relax while I'm sterilizing.
在您活动时请注意尿管。
Be careful with the catheter during any movement.
深静脉置管护理
PICC/Central venous catheter care
我将检查您的深静脉置管。
I am going to check the central venous catheter.
我将对穿刺点进行消毒，请保持不动。
Please hold still while I'm sterilizing the puncture site.
接下来我将为您更换敷贴。
Next, I am going to replace the plaster.

第九章　常用药物及医疗耗材

抗病毒药物

抗病毒	Antiviral
瑞德西韦	Remdesivir
洛匹那韦－利托那韦	Lopinavir-ritonavir
奥司他韦	Oseltamivir
利巴韦林	Ribavirin
阿比多尔	Arbidol
氯喹	Chloroquine
磷酸氯喹	Chloroquine phosphate
羟氯喹	Hydroxychloroquine
干扰素	Interferon

抗菌治疗

抗生素	Antibiotics
广谱抗生素	Broad-spectrum antibiotics
菌群失调	Dysbacteriosis
经验性抗菌治疗	Empirical antibiotic therapy
β内酰胺酶	Beta-lactamase
降阶梯治疗	De-escalation therapy
耐药性	Drug resistance
抗生素敏感	Antibiotic sensitivity (or susceptibility)
青霉素类	Penicillin
阿莫西林	Amoxicillin
阿莫西林克拉维酸钾	Amoxicillin and clavulanate potassium

广谱青霉素	Extended spectrum penicillin
哌拉西林他唑巴坦	Piperacillin and tazobactam
头孢菌素	Cephalosporins
头孢曲松	Ceftriaxone
头孢他啶	Ceftazidime
头孢哌酮钠舒巴坦钠（舒普深）	Cefoperazone sodium and sulbactam sodium (Sulperazone)
头孢呋辛	Cefuroxime
头孢西丁	Cefoxitin
头孢美唑	Cefmetazole
克林霉素	Clindamycin
喹诺酮类	Quinolone
氟喹诺酮	Fluoroquinolone
左氧氟沙星	Levofloxacin
莫西沙星	Moxifloxacin
阿奇霉素	Azithromycin
庆大霉素	Gentamicin
碳青霉烯类	Carbapenem
亚胺培南	Imipenem
美罗培南	Meropenem
帕尼培南	Panipenem
厄他培南	Ertapenem
比阿培南	Biapenem
万古霉素	Vancomycin
替加环素	Tigecycline

利奈唑胺	Linezolid
氨曲南	Aztreonam
甲硝唑	Metronidazole, MNZ
替硝唑	Tinidazole
奥硝唑	Ornidazole
复方新诺明	Sulfamethoxazole and trimethoprim, SMZ-TMP

抗真菌药物

两性霉素 B	Amphotericin B
伏立康唑	Voriconazole
卡泊芬净	Caspofungin
棘白菌素	Echinocandin

抗寄生虫药物

阿苯达唑	Albendazole

被动免疫药物

破伤风抗毒素	Tetanus antitoxin
破伤风免疫球蛋白	Tetanus immune globulin
抗蛇毒血清	Antivenom
狂犬病免疫球蛋白	Rabies immune globulin

解热镇痛药物

解热药物	Antipyretic
镇痛药物	Analgesics

阿片类药物	Opioids
对乙酰氨基酚	Acetaminophen, APAP
非甾体类抗炎药物	Non-steroidal anti-inflammatory drugs, NSAIDs
阿司匹林	Aspirin
吲哚美辛	Indomethacin
萘普生	Naproxen
布洛芬	Ibuprofen
氟比洛芬酯	Flurbiprofen
栓剂	Suppository
哌替啶（杜冷丁）	Pethidine (Dolantin)
吗啡	Morphine
地佐辛	Dezocine

呼吸系统用药

氨溴索（沐舒坦）	Ambroxol (Mucosolvan)
多索茶碱	Doxofylline
沙丁胺醇	Salbutamol
布地奈德混悬剂	Budesonide nebulizer suspension
吸入用异丙托溴铵	Ipratropium bromide
孟鲁司特	Montelukast
乙酰半胱氨酸	Acetylcysteine
止咳药物	Antitussive

心血管系统用药

降压药	Antihypertensive

硝苯地平缓释片	Nifedipine sustained release tablet
尼卡地平（佩尔）	Nicardipine (Perdipine)
地尔硫䓬	Diltiazem
普奈洛尔	Propranolol
美托洛尔（倍他乐克）	Metoprolol (Betaloc)
缬沙坦	Valsartan
厄贝沙坦	Irbesartan
硝酸甘油	Nitroglycerin
硝普钠	Sodium nitroprusside，SNP
洋地黄类	Digitalis
地高辛	Digoxin
肾上腺素	Epinephrine
血管加压药物	Vasopressor
去甲肾上腺素	Norepinephrine
多巴胺	Dopamine
间羟胺（阿拉明）	Metaraminol
血管收缩剂	Vasoconstrictor

消化系统用药

益生菌	Probiotics
质子泵抑制剂	Proton pump inhibitor, PPI
奥美拉唑	Omeprazole
泮托拉唑	Pantoprazole
护肝药	Liver-protective drugs
复方甘草酸单胺	Compound glycyrrhizin

异甘草酸镁	Magnesium isoglycyrrhizinate
甘草酸二铵	Diammonium glycyrrhizinate
止吐药物	Antiemetics
止泻药物	Antidiarrheal
胃肠动力药	Prokinetic drugs

内分泌系统用药

二甲双胍	Metformin
吡格列酮	Pioglitazone
长效胰岛素	Long-acting insulins
甘精胰岛素	Insulin glargine
阿卡波糖	Acarbose
左旋甲状腺素	Levothyroxine
糖皮质激素	Glucocorticoids
琥珀酰氢化可的松	Hydrocortisone sodium succinate
甲基强的松	Methylprednisolone
地塞米松	Dexamethasone

其他常用药物

抗组胺药物	Antihistamine
异丙嗪（非那根）	Promethazine (Phenergan)
苯海拉明	Diphenhydramine
氯雷他定	Loratadine
抗凝药物	Anticoagulant
普通肝素	Heparin
低分子肝素	Low-molecular-weight heparin, LMWH

华法林	Warfarin
氯吡格雷	Clopidogrel
双嘧达莫(潘生丁)	Dipyridamole （Persantine)
利尿药物	Diuretics
呋塞米	Furosemide
托拉塞米	Torasemide
螺内酯	Spironolactone
精神系统药物	Psychotropic drugs
氟哌啶醇	Haloperidol
加巴喷丁	Gabapentin
阿普唑仑	Alprazolam
地西泮	Diazepam
奥氮平	Olanzapine
托珠单抗	Tocilizumab
芬太尼	Fentanyl
肌松药	Muscle relaxant
莫匹罗星	Mupirocin
妥布霉素滴眼液	Ophthalmic tobramycin
红细胞悬液	Erythrocyte suspension
阻断剂 / 拮抗剂	Antagonist

医嘱用法

口服	By mouth / po
吸入	Inhalation
一天 1 次	Once daily / qd
一天 2 次	Twice daily / bid

一天 3 次	Three times a day / tid
一天 4 次	Four times a day / qid
每小时 1 次	Every hour / qh
每 4 小时 1 次	Every four hours / q4h
每晚 1 次	Every evening / qn
每晨 1 次	Every morning / qm
饭前（给药）	Before meal / ac
饭后（给药）	With meal / pc
临睡时	Before bedtime/ hs
需要时（限用一次，12 小时内有效）	When needed / sos
必要时（长期）	When necessary / prn
即刻	Now / st
禁忌证	Contraindications

常用耗材

管材类	Tube / Catheter
吸痰管	Suction catheter
鼻导管	Nasal tube
鼻氧管	Nasal oxygen tube
输氧管	Oxygen supply tube
鼻胃管	Nasogastric tube
喂食管	Feeding tube
导尿管	Forley catheter
气管导管	Tracheal tube
气管切开导管	Tracheostomy tube

面罩类	Mask
氧气面罩	Oxygen mask
雾化面罩	Nebulizer mask
普通面罩	Standard mask
文丘里面罩	Venturi mask
储氧面罩	Non-rebreather mask, NRB
球囊面罩 / 简易呼吸器	Bag-Valve-Mask, BVM
绷带类	Bandage
弹力绷带	Elastic bandage
纱布绷带	Gauze bandage
粘性绷带	Cohesive bandage
网状弹力绷带	Tubular net bandage
胶带类	Tape
无纺布胶带	Non-woven tape
纸胶带	Paper tape
弹力黏性胶带	Elastic adhesive tape
一次性输液敷贴	Disposable infusion plaster
纱布类	Gauze
无纺布纱布片	Non-woven gauze
脱脂纱布	Absorbent cotton gauze
敷料类	Dressing
创口贴	Adhesive wound plaster
眼贴	Eye pad
棉球	Cotton ball
脱脂药棉	Absorbent cotton wool

耗材类	Consumables
一次性的	Disposable
注射器	Syringe
延长管	Extension tube
三通阀	Three-way stopcock
肝素帽	Heparin cap
针头	Needle
头皮静脉留置针	Scalp vein indwelling needle
留置针	Indwelling needle
采血针	Blood lancet
静脉注射	Intravenous injection
输液器	Infusion set
输血器	Blood transfusion set
胰岛素注射器	Insulin syringe
胰岛素笔针	Insulin pen needle
安瓿	Ampule
吊篮（挂袋）	Hanger
输液袋	Infusion bag
输液管	Infusion tube
输液架	Infusion stand
吸痰器	Mucus extractor
管饲器	Feeding syringe
冲洗器 / 灌注器	Irrigation syringe
外科缝合线	Surgical suture
手术帽	Surgical cap
护士帽	Nurse cap

手术衣	Surgical gown
隔离服	Isolation gown
鞋套	Shoe cover
压舌板	Tongue depressor
急救包	First-aid kit
尿袋	Urine bag
酒精棉球	Alcohol swab
棉签	Q-tips
冰袋	Ice bag/pack
听诊器	Stethoscope
体温计	Thermometer
血压袖带	Blood pressure cuff
剪刀	Scissors
取样器皿	Specimen container
带尺	Measuring tape
药杯	Medicine cup
水杯	Water cup
床旁桌	Bedside table
床栏	Bedside rails
床帘	Curtain
吸管	Straw
餐具	Utensil
餐叉	Fork
餐刀	Knife
托盘	Tray
尿壶	Urinal

盆	Basin
餐巾纸	Napkin
纸巾	Tissue
擦手纸	Paper towel
湿纸巾	Wipes
便盆	Bedpan
便桶	Commode
牙膏	Toothpaste
牙刷	Toothbrush
漱口水	Mouth wash
卫生巾	Pad
卫生棉条	Tampon
床上垫料	Bed pads
尿不湿	Diaper
浴巾	Bath towel
床垫	Mattress
枕头	Pillow
枕套	Pillowcase
床上用品	Linen
毯子	Blanket
患者转移板	Patient transfer sheet
患者私人物品	Patient personal stuff

／第十章　医疗流程及院感防控／

流行病学 / 病源追溯

流行病学	Epidemiology
流行病学调查	Epidemiological investigation
始发症状	Initial symptom
传染性的	Contagious / Communicable
易感人群	Vulnerable population
暴发	Outbreak
感染地点 / 事件	Infection place / event
当地	Local
疫区	Affected area
聚餐	Dine together
聚集 / 集会	Gathering
聚集病例	Cluster cases
联防联控机制	Joint prevention and control mechanism
健康申报	Declaration of health
地方性流行病	Endemic disease
流行性传染病	Epidemic disease
全球大流行	Pandemic disease
公共场所	Public places
暴露程度	Exposure status
暴露	Exposure
潜在暴露	Potential exposure
密切接触	Close contact
直接接触	Direct contact

传播途径	Transmission route
飞沫传播	Droplet transmission
空气传播	Airborne transmission
人传人	Human-to-human transmission
社区传播	Community transmission
当地传播	Local transmission
预防与干预	Precaution and intervention
社会距离	Social distancing
社区干预	Community intervention
集中隔离	Quarantine at assembly site
居家隔离	Stay-at-home policy
自我隔离	Self-isolation
单间隔离	Single room isolation
自我监测	Self-monitoring
手卫生	Hand hygiene
流感疫苗	Flu shot

预检分诊

分诊	Triage
分诊区	Triage area
红外体温计	Infrared thermometer
水银体温计	Mercury thermometer
筛查	Screen
门诊	Outpatient
医疗服务	Medical service
急诊	Emergent / Urgent care clinic

紧急医疗服务	Emergency medical service, EMS
住院患者	Inpatient
重症监护	Critical care
就诊者分类	Patients classification
受检人员	Persons under inspection, PUI
潜伏期	Incubation period
疑似患者	Suspected patient
有症状患者	Symptomatic patient
无症状患者	Asymptomatic patient
确诊病例	Confirmed case
高危患者	High-risk patient
预后相关	Prognosis
危急	Critical
致命	Fatal
重症	Severe
恶化	Deterioration
致死	Fatality
合并症	Comorbidity
死亡率	Mortality
康复	Recovery

院感防控措施

院感防控	Hospital infection prevention
检疫隔离	Quarantine
疏散	Evacuation
防控区	Areas for prevention and control

隔离观察区	Quarantine area
清洁区	Clean area
潜在污染区	Potentially contaminated area
缓冲区	Buffer area / Doffing area
污染区	Contaminated area
负压病房	Negative pressure ward
通道	Passageway
单间	Separate room
患者转运	Patient transfer
转运	Transfer
担架	Stretcher
负压担架	Negative pressure stretcher
单进	One-way entrance
单出	One-way exit
门禁	Access control
指定路线	Designated route
预防措施	Precautions
飞沫传播预防措施	Droplet precautions
接触传播预防措施	Contact precautions
空气传播预防措施	Airborne precautions
消毒	Disinfect
终末消毒	Terminal disinfection
通风良好	Well-ventilated

环境消杀

环境消杀	Environmental cleaning & disinfection

交叉感染	Cross-infection
生物危害废物	Biohazardous waste
有感染性的物品	Infectious materials
被污染的医疗物品	Contaminated medical supplies
物体表面	Surfaces of an object
被污染的空气	Contaminated air
气溶胶	Aerosol
体液	Body fluid
分泌物	Secretions
粪便	Stool
消毒剂	Disinfectant
含氯消毒剂	Chlorine disinfectant
含醇手部消毒剂	Alcohol-based hand rub, ABHR
乙醇	Ethanol
氯己定	Chlorhexidine
漂白剂	Bleach
洗涤剂	Detergent
洗手液	Hand sanitizer
空气消毒机	Air sterilizer
高效空气过滤器	High-efficiency particulate air (HEPA) filter
空气传播隔离病房	Airborne infection isolation rooms, AIIRs

第十一章　常用医学缩略词

A		
A & W	Alive and Well	活着且健康
Ab	Antibody	抗体
ABC	Aspiration Biopsy Cytology	针吸活检细胞学
ABD	Abdomen	腹部
ac	Ante Cibum	饭前（给药）
ACE	Angiotensin Converting Enzyme	血管紧张素转换酶
ACEI	Angiotensin Converting Enzyme Inhibitor	血管紧张素转换酶抑制剂
Ach	Acetylcholine	乙酰胆碱
AD	Alzheimer Disease	阿尔茨海默病
AF	Atrial Fibrillation	房颤
Ag	Antigen	抗原
AGPs	Aerosol-Generating Procedures	产生气溶胶的操作
AIDS	Acquired Immunodeficiency Syndrome	获得性免疫缺陷综合征
ALS	Advanced Life Support	高级生命支持
AMI	Acute Myocardial Infarction	急性心肌梗塞
AML	Acute Myeloblastic (Myelogenous) Leukemia	急性髓系白血病
ANS	Autonomic Nervous System	自主神经系统
AP	Antero-Posterior	前后位
APAP	Acetaminophen	对乙酰氨基酚

ARB	Angiotensin Receptor Blocker	血管紧张素受体拮抗剂
ARDS	Acute Respiratory Distress Syndrome	急性呼吸窘迫综合征
ARF	Acute Respiratory Failure	急性呼吸衰竭
ASAP	As soon as possible	尽快
ATP	Adenosine Triphosphate	腺苷三磷酸
AXR	Abdominal X-Ray	腹部 X 光片
B		
BAL	Bronchoalveolar Lavage (fluid)	支气管肺泡灌洗液
bid	Bis In Die	一天 2 次
BM	Bowel Movement	排便
BMI	Body Mass Index	体重指数
BMR	Basic Metabolic Rate	基本代谢率
BMT	Bone Mineral Density	骨密度
BP	Blood Pressure	血压
bpm	Beats per Minute	每分搏动次数
BSA	Body Surface Area	体表面积
BT	Bleeding Time	出血时间
C		
C/F	Chill / Fever	寒颤 / 发热
C/o	Complain of	主诉
CA	Cancer	癌症
CABG	Coronary Artery Bypass Graft	冠状动脉搭桥术
CAD	Coronary Artery Disease	冠心病
cap	Capsule	胶囊

CBD	Common Bile Duct	胆总管
CBF	Cerebral Blood Flow	脑血流量
CBR	Complete Bed Rest	绝对卧床休息
CC	Chief Complaint	主诉
CCB	Calcium Channel Blocker	钙通道阻滞剂
CCM	Continuous Cardiac Monitoring	持续心电监护
CCPD	Continuous Cyclic Peritoneal Dialysis	持续循环式腹膜透析
CHD	Coronary Heart Disease	冠心病
CNS	Central Nervous System	中枢神经系统
CO_2	Carbon Dioxide	二氧化碳
CO_2cp	Carbon Dioxide Combining Power	二氧化碳结合力
COLD	Chronic Obstructive Lung Disease	慢性阻塞性肺疾病
COPD	Chronic Obstructive Pulmonary Disease	慢性阻塞性肺疾病
COX-2	Cyclooxygenase-2	环氧化酶 -2
CPAP	Continuous Positive Airway Pressure	持续气道正压
CPR	Cardiopulmonary Resuscitation	心肺复苏
CPT	Chest Physical Treatment	胸部物理治疗
Cr	Creatinine	肌酐
CRF	Chronic Renal Failure	慢性肾衰
CRRT	Continuous Renal Replacement Therapy	连续性肾脏替代治疗
CSF	Cerebrospinal Fluid	脑脊液
CSII	Continuous Subcutaneous Insulin Infusion	胰岛素持续皮下输注

CT	Computed Tomograpy	电子计算机断层扫描
CTA	CT Angiography	CT 血管造影
CVA	Cerebrovascular Accident	脑血管意外
CVD	Cardiovascular Disease	心血管疾病
CVI	Chronic Venous Insufficiency	慢性静脉功能不全
CVP	Central Venous Pressure	中心静脉压
CXR	Chest X-Ray	胸部 X 光片
D		
D & V	Diarrhoea and Vomiting	腹泻、呕吐
D/C	Discontinue	停药
D/H	Drug History	用药史
DBP	Diastolic Blood Pressure	舒张压
DIC	Disseminated Intravascular Coagulation	弥漫性血管内凝血
DM	Diabetes Mellitus	糖尿病
DNA	Deoxyribonucleic Acid	脱氧核糖核酸
DOB	Date of Birth	出生日期
Dr.	Doctor	医生，博士
DVT	Deep Vein Thrombosis	深静脉血栓
Dx	Diagnosis	诊断
E		
EBV	Epstein-Barr Virus	EB 病毒
ECG	Electrocardiogram	心电图
ECMO	Extracorporeal Membrane Oxygenation	体外膜肺氧合
EEG	Electroencephalography	脑电图

EGD	Esophago-Gastroduodenoscopy	食管—胃十二指肠镜检查
ELISA	Enzyme-Linked Immunosorbent Assay	酶联免疫吸附试验
Enem.	Enema	灌肠剂
ER	Endoplasmic Reticulum	内质网
ER	Emergency Room	急诊室
ERV	Expiratory Reserve Volume	补呼气量
ESR	Erythrocyte Sedimentation Rate	红细胞沉降率
ESRD	End-Stage Renal Disease	终末期肾病
ETA	Estimated Time of Arrival	预计到达时间
EtOH	Ethyl Alcohol	酒精
F		
F°	Fahrenheit Temperature	华氏温度
FAQ	Frequently Asked Questions	常见问答
FBC	Full Blood Count	全血计数
FBG	Fasting Blood Glucose	空腹血糖
FBS	Fasting Blood Sugar	空腹血糖
FDA	Food and Drug Administration	食品药品监督管理局
FEV	Forced Expiratory Volume	用力呼气量
FFP	Fresh Frozen Plasma	新鲜冰冻血浆
FH	Family History	家族史
FiO_2	Fraction of inspired oxygen	吸氧浓度
FMS	Fibromyalgia Syndrome	纤维肌痛综合征
FRC	Functional Residual Capacity	功能残气量
FUO	Fever of Unknown Origin	不明原因发热

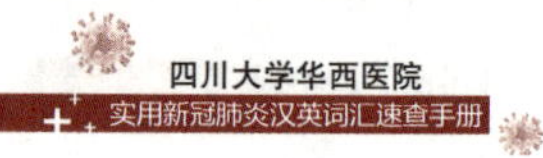

FVC	Forced Vital Capacity	用力肺活量
FYI	For Your Information	供你参考
G		
GCS	Glasgow Coma Scale	格拉斯哥昏迷评分
GFR	Glomerular Filtration Rate	肾小球滤过率
GI	Gastrointestinal	胃肠道
Gm–	Gram-Negative	革兰阴性
Gm+	Gram-Positive	革兰阳性
GU	Genitourinary	泌尿生殖的
H		
H & P	History and Physical Examination	病史和体格检查
h/o	History of...	……病史
HAV	Hepatitis A Virus	甲型肝炎病毒
Hb	Hemoglobin	血红蛋白
HBV	Hepatitis B Virus	乙型肝炎病毒
HCl	Hydrochloric Acid	盐酸
HCTZ	Hydrochlorothiazide	氢氯噻嗪
HCV	Hepatitis C Virus	丙型肝炎病毒
HDV	Hepatitis D Virus	丁型肝炎病毒
HEV	Hepatitis E Virus	戊型肝炎病毒
HFNC	High-Flow Nasal Cannula	高流量鼻导管
HI	Head Injury	头部伤害
HIV	Human Immunodeficiency Virus	人类免疫缺陷病毒
HNPU	Has Not Passed Urine	未排尿
HPI	History of Present Illness	现病史
HPV	Human Papillomavirus	人乳头瘤病毒

HR	Heart Rate	心率
hs	Hora Somni	临睡前
Ht	Height	身高
HTN	Hypertension	高血压
Hx	History	病史
Hz	Hertz	赫兹
I		
I & D	Incision and Drainage	切开引流
I / O	Intake and Output	出入量
IABP	Intraaortic Balloon Pump	主动脉内气囊泵
IBD –	Inflammatory Bowel Disease	炎症性肠病
IBS –	Inflammatory Bowel Syndrome	炎性肠道综合征
IC	Inspiratory Capacity	最大吸气量
ICH	Intracerebral Hemorrhage	脑出血
ICP	Intracranial Pressure	颅内压
ICU	Intensive Care Unit	重症监护室
ID	Intradermal	经皮
ID	Infectious Disease	感染性疾病
IF	Intrinsic Factor	内因子
IFG	Impaired Fasting Glucose	空腹血糖受损
Ig	Immunoglobulins	免疫球蛋白
IGRA	Interferon-Gamma Release Assay	干扰素释放反应
IGT	Impaired Glucose Tolerance	糖耐量受损
IHSS	Idiopathic Hypertrophic Subaortic Stenosis	特发性肥厚性主动脉瓣下狭窄
IM	Intramuscular	经肌肉

Inj.	Injection Fluid	注射剂
INH	Isoniazid	异烟肼
IOP	Intra-Ocular Pressure	眼内压
IPPA	Inspection, Palpation, Percussion, Auscultation	视触叩听
IPPV	Intermittent Positive Pressure Ventilation	间歇正压通气
IRV	Inspiratory Reserve Volume	补吸气量
ITP	Idiopathic Thrombocytopenic Purpura	特发性血小板减少性紫癜
IV	Intravenous	经静脉
IVDA	Intravenous Drug Abuse	静脉注射药物滥用
ivgtt	Intravenous Drip	静脉滴注
In vivo	In the Body	体内
In vitro	Outside the Living body	体外
L		
LE	Lupus Erythematosus	红斑狼疮
LFT	Liver Function Test	肝功能检查
LL	Left Lateral	左侧位
LLQ	Left Lower Quadrant	左下腹
LN	Lymph Node	淋巴结
LOC	Level of Consciousness	意识水平
LP	Lumbar Puncture	腰椎穿刺
LUL	Left Upper Lobe	左上叶
LUQ	Left Upper Quadrant	左上腹
LV	Left Ventricle	左心室

LVDD	Left Ventricular Diastolic Dysfunction	左心室舒张功能障碍
LVEDP	Left Ventricular End-Diastolic Pressure	左心室舒张末压
LVH	Left Ventricular Hypertrophy	左心室肥厚
LVSD	Left Ventricular Systolic Dysfunction	左心室收缩功能不全
M		
MAOI	Monoamine Oxidase Inhibitor	单胺氧化酶抑制剂
MAP	Mean Arterial Pressure	平均动脉压
MCV	Mean Corpuscular Volume	平均红细胞体积
Med. Rec#	Medical Record Number	病历号
MEFR	Maximal Expiratory Flow Rate	最大呼气流速
MEN	Multiple Endocrine Neoplasia	多样内分泌瘤
MG	Myasthenia Gravis	重症肌无力
MI	Myocardial Infarction	心肌梗塞
mL	Milliliter	毫升
mm Hg	Millimeters of Mercury	毫米汞柱
MMFR	Maximum Midexpiratory Flow Rate	最大呼气中段流率
MMT	Manual Muscle Test	肌力检查
MRI	Magnetic Resonance Imaging	核磁共振成像
MRSA	Methicillin-Resistant *Staphylococcus Aureus*	耐甲氧西林金黄色葡萄球菌
MSE	Mental State Examination	精神状态检查
MSU	Mid-Stream Urine	中段尿

MTB	*Mycobacterium Tuberculosis*	结核分枝杆菌
N		
N/A	Non-Apply	不需要
N/S	Normal Saline	生理盐水
NAD	No Apparent Distress	无明显不适
NG	Nasogastric	鼻胃管
NICU	Neonatal Intensive Care Unit	新生儿重症监护病房
NIH	National Institutes of Health	国家卫生研究院
NKA	Non-Known Allergies	无已知的过敏史
NKDA	No Known Drug Allergies	无已知的药物过敏史
NPH	Normal Pressure Hydrocephalus	正常压力性脑积水
NPO	Nothing by Mouth	禁食
NSAIDs	Nonsteroidal Antiinflammatory Drugs	非甾体类抗炎药物
NSFW	Not Safe for Work	不适合工作场所
NSTEMI	Non-ST Elevation Myocardial Infarction	非 ST 段抬高的心肌梗塞
O		
OB	Occult Blood	隐血
o.d.	Once a Day	一天 1 次
OGTT	Oral Glucose Tolerance Test	口服糖耐量试验
OOB	Out of Bed	下床
OT	Occupational Therapy	作业疗法
OTC	Over-the-Counter	非处方药
OUI	Overflow Urine Incontinence	溢出性尿失禁

P		
P.	Pulse	脉搏
PA	Physician Assistant	医师助理
PA	Postero-Anterior	后前位
PACU	Postanesthesia Care Unit	麻醉后恢复室
PAP	Pulmonary Arterial Pressure	肺动脉压力
Past.	Paste	糊剂
pc	Post Cibum	饭后（给药）
PCA	Patient-Controlled Analgesia	患者自控镇痛
PCWP	Pulmonary Capillary Wedge Pressure	肺毛细血管楔压
PE	Physical Examination	体格检查
PE	Pulmonary Embolism	肺栓塞
PE	Pleural Effusion	胸腔积液
PEEP	Positive End-Expiratory Pressure	呼气末正压
PEP	Protein Electrophoresis	蛋白电泳
PET	Positron Emission Tomography	正电子发射计算机断层扫描
PFT	Pulmonary Function Test	肺功能检查
PICC	Peripherally Inserted Central Catheter	经外周中心静脉置管
PIP	Peak Inspiratory Pressure	吸气峰压
PMH	Past Medical History	既往病史
PND	Paroxysmal Nocturnal Dyspnea	夜间阵发性呼吸困难
PNS	Peripheral Nervous System	外周神经系统
po	Per Os	口服
Postop.	Postoperative	术后

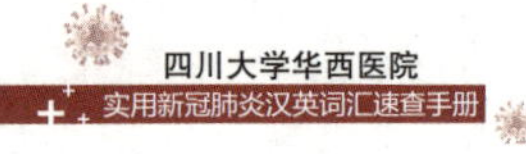

pp	Postprandial (After A Meal)	饭后
PPD	Purified Protein Derivative	结核菌素纯蛋白衍生物
PPE	Personal Protective Equipment	个人防护用品
PPI	Proton Pump Inhibitor	质子泵抑制剂
Preop.	Preoperative	术前
prn	Pro Re Nata	按需
PSA	Prostate-Specific Antigen	前列腺特异性抗原
PUI	Paradoxical Urinary Incontinence	反常性尿失禁
Q		
q4h	Quaque Quarta Hora	每 4 小时 1 次
qam	Quaque Ante Meridiem	每个早晨
qd	Quaque Die	一天 1 次
qh	Quaque Hora	每小时 1 次
qid	Quater In Die	一天 4 次
qm	Quaque Mane	每晨 1 次
qn	Quaque Nocte	每晚 1 次
qp	Quaque Hora	每小时
R		
RA	Rheumatoid Arthritis	类风湿性关节炎
RDS	Respiratory Distress Syndrome	呼吸窘迫综合征
RL	Right Lateral	右侧位
RLQ	Right Lower Quadrant	右下腹
RML	Right Middle Lobe	右肺中叶
RMT	Respiratory Muscle Training	呼吸肌锻炼

RNA	Ribonucleic Acid	核糖核酸
ROM	Range of Motion	活动范围
ROS	Review of Systems	系统回顾
RR	Respiratory Rate	呼吸频率
RR	Respiration Rhythm	呼吸节律
RSV	Respiratory Syncytial Virus	呼吸道合胞病毒
RT	Reverse Transcription	逆转录
RTC	Rotator Cuff	旋转袖
RUQ	Right Upper Quadrant	右上腹
RV	Residual Volume	残气量
RX	Drug prescription	处方
S		
S/S	Signs and Symptoms	体征和症状
SAB	Spontaneous Abortion	自发性流产
SARS	Severe Acute Respiratory Syndrome	严重急性呼吸综合征
SBO	Small Bowel Obstruction	小肠梗阻
SBP	Systolic Blood Pressure	收缩压
SC	Subcutaneous	皮下
SL	Sublingual	舌下
SOB	Shortness of Breath	呼吸短促
SOS	Si Opus Sit	必要时只用 1 次
SPECT	Single-Photon Emission Computed Tomography	单光子发射计算机断层扫描
st.	Statim	即刻
Staph.	Staphylococcus	葡萄球菌

STEMI	ST- Elevation Myocardial Infarction	ST 段抬高的心肌梗塞
Strep.	Streptococcus	链球菌
Sx	Symptoms	症状
T		
T	Temperature	体温
T1DM	Type 1 Diabetes Mellitus	I 型糖尿病
T2DM	Type 2 Diabetes Mellitus	Ⅱ型糖尿病
TB	Tuberculosis	结核
TCO_2	Total Carbon Dioxide	二氧化碳总量
TEE	Transesophageal Echocardiogram	经食道超声
tid	Ter In Die	一天 3 次
TLC	Total Lung Capacity	肺容量
TNM	Tumor-Lymph Node-Metastasis	肿瘤－淋巴结转移
tPA	Tissue Plasminogen Activator	组织型纤溶酶原激活物
TPN	Total Parenteral Nutrition	全肠外营养
TTP	Thrombotic Thrombocytopenic Purpura	血栓性血小板减少性紫癜
TV	Tidal Volume	潮气量
U		
UA	Urinalysis	尿液分析
UAO	Upper Airway Obstruction	上气道梗阻
Ung.	Unguent	软膏剂
URI	Upper Respiratory Infection	上呼吸道感染
US	Ultrasound	超声

UTI	Urinary Tract Infection	尿路感染
V		
VC	Vital Capacity	肺活量
VF	Ventricular Fibrillation	心室颤动
VRSA	Vancomycin-Resistant *Staphylococcus Aureus*	耐万古霉素金黄色葡萄球菌
VS	Vital Signs	生命体征
VT	Ventricular Tachycardia	室性心动过速
VTE	Venous Thromboembolism	静脉血栓栓塞
W		
w/o	Without	没有
Y		
y/o	...years old	……岁